ADAPTIVE SPATIAL ALIGNMENT

SCIENTIFIC PSYCHOLOGY SERIES

Monographs

Edited Volumes

ADAPTIVE SPATIAL ALIGNMENT

Gordon M. Redding
Illinois State University

Benjamin Wallace
Cleveland State University

LEA

LAWRENCE ERLBAUM ASSOCIATES, PUBLISHERS
1997   Mahwah, New Jersey

Lawrence Erlbaum Associates, Inc., Publishers
10 Industrial Avenue
Mahwah, New Jersey 07430

Library of Congress Cataloging-In-Publication Data

Redding, Gordon M.
Adaptive Spatial Alignment/ Gordon M. Redding, Benjamin
Wallace.
       p. cm.
    Includes bibliographical references and indexes.
    ISBN 0-8058-2395-6 (alk. paper)
    1. Space perception. 2. Adaptation (Physiology) 3.
Prisms. 4. Perceptual–motor learning. I. Wallace, Ben-
jamin. II. Title
    QP443.R43 1997
    153.7'54—DC20   96-41210
                                CIP

Printed in the United States of America
10 9 8 7 6 5 4 3 2 1

TABLE OF CONTENTS

PREFACE

For most people, prism adaptation is an amusing demonstration, first experienced perhaps in an introductory psychology course. When we wear goggles containing prisms that optically displace the visual field, we make dramatic errors in, for example, throwing a ball. Our performance, however, rapidly improves, and, when the prisms are removed, we make throwing errors in the opposite direction! For those of us who have spent a substantial part of our academic careers investigating prism adaptation, it has been a challenging puzzle to understand how the phenomenon fits in with the rest of cognitive science. This monograph relates this peculiar phenomenon to the larger context of cognitive science, especially motor control and learning. This monograph is not only about prism adaptation, but so much more.

The three chapters of Part I, Perceptual–Motor Performance, sketch the background concepts necessary to understand the contribution of prism adaptation to the larger issue of adaptive perceptual–motor performance. Chapter 1, Strategic Perceptual–Motor Control, reviews the basic concepts of motor control and learning that enable strategic response in the prism adaptation situation. Chapter 2, Sensorimotor Transformation, develops a hypothesis about spatial representation and spatial mapping and introduces the basic idea of adaptive spatial alignment. Chapter 3, Perceptual–Motor Learning, contrasts perceptual and motor learning and reviews evidence for the involvement of nonassociative and associative learning in prism adaptation.

The four chapters of Part II, Prism Adaptation, are directly concerned with data and theory in prism adaptation. Chapter 4, Paradigm and Generalizations, outlines prism adaptation methodology and lists several empirical conclusions from previous research that constrained development of the theoretical framework presented in the next two chapters. Chapter 5, Contributions of Strategic Control, presents a theory of strategic perceptual–motor control and learning that enables adaptive performance during prism exposure, but which does not directly involve adaptive spatial alignment. Chapter 6, Alignment and Realignment, extends the theory to include realignment processes that correct for the spatial misalignment among sensorimotor systems produced by prisms. Chapter 7, Theoretical Issues, shows how traditional issues in prism adaptation may be rephrased in terms of the present theoretical framework.

In the three chapters of Part III, Research, we review the research we have conducted in developing and testing the present theory of prism adaptation. Chapter 8, Adaptation During Locomotion, summarizes our initial investigations employing a naturalistic exposure setting and chapter 9, Adaptive Eye–Hand Coordination, reports some more rigorous tests with an experimentally constrained research paradigm. Chapter 10, Implications, points out the more general theoretical issues raised by our analysis of prism adaptation and makes specific suggestions for further research within the prism adaptation paradigm.

Throughout this effort, we have been guided by the conviction that prism adaptation cannot be understood within a narrow context and, moreover, that prism adaptation research has broad implications for adaptive perceptual–motor performance. We believe this monograph establishes the prism adaptation paradigm as a major tool for research and theory development.

Development of the view of prism adaptation presented in this monograph was begun while the first author was a visiting professor (1982–1983) in the Department of Psychology at the University of Oregon. He gratefully acknowledges the courtesies and facilities extended to him at that time. The authors also appreciate the constructive comments from Brian Craske, Elizabeth Rodriguez, Yves Rossetti, Bob Welch, and Dan Willingham on earlier versions of this manuscript. We especially wish to acknowledge Bob Welch's (1978) review of the prism adaptation literature. Without this extensive review of research the present work would not have been possible. Also, Felice Bedford's fundamental insight (e.g., 1989) into the nature of learning filled a large gap in our thinking about prism adaptation.

We owe an immeasurable debt to our many students (and sometimes coauthors). Without their assistance in the laboratory and the intellectual stimulation they provided, the research base for this monograph simply would not have happened. We hope that the following list is complete: Bruce Anderson, Diane Anspach, Albert Borroni, Susan Carlisle, Steve Clark, Daniel Collier, Dan Covey, James Cummins, Douglas Freud, Rob Hitlan, Bruce Kelsay, Don Lucas, Ian Lucash, Sondra Patterson, Jodi Penwell, Mary Persanyi, Steve Rader, Gabe Radvansky, David Swift, Mary Swift, Deanna Turosky, and Jenifer Waisure.

We are especially grateful to our respective departments for their support and encouragement of obscure research programs that garner little external funding. Departmental technical personnel (Dennis Householder, Jeff Imig, and Don Meiser) are also deserving of our thanks. We hope our mentors in prism adaptation (Shelly Ebenholtz, Bill Epstein, and Larry Melamed) find this work satisfactory. They share the credit, but not the responsibility. To the many reviewers of our manuscripts (especially Felice Bedford, Digby Elliott, and Yves Rossetti), we are grateful for the sometimes painful but always constructive advice.

The many conversations with Larry Erlbaum over the years during which the ideas expressed here took shape encouraged our dream of seeing these ideas in print. And the competence of the editorial staff at Lawrence Erlbaum Associates made the dream real. We are especially grateful for Judi Amsel's unfailing enthusiasm. Our thanks also go to the Series editors, Steve Link and Jim Townsend, whose editorial comments enabled improvements in the manuscript.

No list of acknowledgments would be complete without recognition of support from our families, especially Donna Redding. Her faith in the quality of our work and encouragement (not to say prodding) of her husband assured timely development of the manuscript.

PART I

PERCEPTUAL–MOTOR PERFORMANCE

The subjective ease of perceptual–motor performance belies the enormous complexity of the underlying integrative apparatus. Even simple actions like rotating a wristwatch into view or reaching for a coffee cup require integration of thousands of sensors, neurons, and motor units. The computational complexity is compounded by the fact that actions can be strategically varied to accommodate different circumstances. For instance, rotating a wristwatch into view when the hand is firmly grasping a steering wheel must be done differently than when the hand is hanging loosely at one's side, and retrieving a coffee cup from a cluttered desk is different from grabbing a cup from a cleared countertop. Obviously, considerable thinking must be accomplished to enable successful perceptual–motor performance even for simple tasks. Theories of perceptual–motor performance characterize such strategies in terms of trajectory planning and feedback control.

The challenge to understanding perceptual–motor performance becomes even more intimidating when we realize that the various perceptual and motor elements do not speak the same language. For instance, perceptual elements speak in terms of visual coordinates and limb angles, but motor elements ultimately only understand muscle lengths and tensions. Obviously, much translating must be done to enable even simple perceptual–motor actions. Theories of perceptual–motor performance conceptualize this process as one of transformations (translations) among the various informational representations (languages).

We also must recognize that the various languages employed by constituent perceptual–motor elements are not fixed but change with time, and, consequently, the rules of translation must change. For instance, as a baby grows, limb weight and length increase. The correspondence between a given set of limb angles and muscle lengths and tensions required to achieve that set of angles also changes. A new pair of eyeglasses may also change the relationship between seen hand position and the matching set of limb angles, requiring an adjustment in the transformation between visual and proprioceptive space.

Moreover, as with any natural system, the human brain is subject to wear and tear, natural cell death, which may cause a slow change in correspondence among the various perceptual and motor elements, and brain trauma may exaggerate this

1

process. Obviously, a lot of learning must be continually occurring to enable perceptual–motor transformations. Theories of perceptual–motor performance usually refer to this process of establishing spatial correspondence among the various perceptual and motor elements as calibration.

Research in perceptual–motor performance usually treats the topics of control, transformations, and calibration in an insular fashion. In the three chapters of Part I we attempt an integrative treatment because we believe that prism adaptation phenomena cannot be understood in any other way. In chapter 1, Strategic Perceptual–Motor Control, we lay the groundwork for understanding the strategies that enable rapid adaptive performance during prism exposure but that do not solve the more fundamental problem posed by the prismatic distortion. In chapter 2, Sensorimotor Transformations, we discuss the spatial transformations necessary for intrinsic representations of extrinsic space and develop the idea of spatial alignment in axes and origins of intrinsic coordinate systems, which is disturbed by the common prismatic distortions of rotation and translation. In chapter 3, Perceptual–Motor Learning, we contrast theories of perceptual and motor learning to develop the hypothesis that adaptive spatial alignment is not simply perceptual or motor learning but a distinct kind of perceptual–motor learning.

Chapter 1

STRATEGIC
PERCEPTUAL–MOTOR CONTROL

Research on the adaptability of perceptual–motor performance to artificially induced spatial misalignment suggests that multiple adaptive processes are evoked by the prism adaptation paradigm. We begin by discussing one of these processes, strategic perceptual–motor control.

Under the broad heading of this chapter, we refer to the perceptual and motor processes that comprise a coordination task and that are flexibly recruited to maximize perceptual–motor performance under changing task demands. By strategic we do not mean a restriction to conscious or attentional processing, although we do mean to exclude consideration of learning. Learning in its several varieties are considered in chapter 3.

In this chapter, we consider the various ways in which the perceptual–motor system can maximize performance. Some of these strategies reflect the results of learning, but learning is not involved in their application to a particular task. Some may reflect how the system strategically disposes its various resources within the natural (inherited) structure of the system. *Strategic* is used almost synonymously with *adaptive,* but the term strategic captures the idea that there are multiple ways to behave adaptively and that adaptive behavior involves choice among available ways. We are concerned here with the *skilled* actor.

At the risk of being obvious, we wish to step back and view the perceptual–motor system from the perspective of its strategic flexibility. We realize that this flexibility poses large problems of explanation at the detailed level, but we should not lose sight of the primary goal. Our treatment of strategic perceptual–motor control is heuristic rather than formal, kinematic rather than dynamic, and behavioral rather than neurological. No attempt is made to force a fit with formal control theory. Rather, such concepts are employed heuristically, freely mixed with information processing concepts in such a manner as is guaranteed to make an engineer blush. We hope that such a coarse sketch will point the way to a more refined as well as more formal understanding.

DEGREES OF FREEDOM AND MOTOR EQUIVALENCE

Redundant degrees of freedom of movement and consequential motor equivalence (Hebb, 1949; Lashley, 1930) are fundamental illustrations of strategic flexibility in perceptual–motor performance. An effector system may have a higher dimensionality than the goal specification. For example, as illustrated in the top part of Fig. 1.1, an arm has seven degrees of freedom of movement. Three degrees of freedom are contributed by the shoulder, which can move up or down and side to side and can twist. Two degrees of freedom arise from the ability of the elbow to bend and twist. The final two degrees of freedom are contributed by up or down and side-to-side movement of the wrist.

A path for the finger to reach a target, however, is specified in three-dimensional space. This means that many different spatial paths of the finger from initial to final position are possible. In one sense, all of these paths are equivalent in terms of achieving the target, but some paths may be more effective than others, especially when the system is faced with external constraints like obstacles, as illustrated in the bottom part of Fig. 1.1. Redundant degrees of freedom and motor equivalence are also advantageous when the spatial path is prescribed, but external constraints limit effector freedom of movement. For example, writing can still be achieved in confined places that limit usual joint movement. Thus, motor equivalence is a reflection of flexibility to varying task demands.

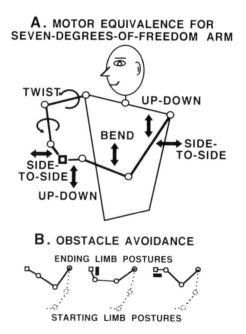

FIG. 1.1.   Motor equivalence and redundant degrees of freedom. A. The arm has seven degrees of freedom of movement: the shoulder can move up and down, side to side and can twist (3); the elbow can bend and twist (2); the wrist can move up and down and side to side (2). A target in three-dimensional space can, therefore, be achieved by many different spatial paths for the limb and different final limb postures. B. Some movement paths and final limb postures are more effective than others, for example, when obstacles are present.

Traditionally, this aspect of perceptual–motor control has been seen as a problem of explanation (Bernstein, 1967). "How does an organism rapidly and correctly choose among the alternative (motor) means than are available to perform spatially defined tasks on different occasions?" (Bullock, Grossberg, & Guenther, 1993, p. 408). One solution to this "degrees of freedom problem" is to suppose that the movement plan incorporates internal constraints designed to produce the most efficient or optimal movement out of all possible movements. For example, constraints have been designed to avoid extreme limb angles (Cruse, 1986), minimize rate of change of acceleration (Hogan & Flash, 1987), and minimize changes in muscle torque (Uno, Kawato, & Suzuki, 1989).

Another approach depends on functional connections among components of the motor system (i.e., synergies) to reduce the degrees of freedom (Bernstein, 1967). The evolutionary history of an organism provides numerous instances in which a collection of joint motions can be synchronously controlled as a single unit. Such synergies have the obvious advantage of reducing the degrees of freedom that must be independently controlled. The idea is that the movement plan incorporates a knowledge of such synergies that internally constrain selection from among all possible movements. For example, synergies have been proposed to exist between angular velocities of elbow and shoulder in terminal reaching movements (Soechting & Lacquaniti, 1981), between eye and hand movements in pointing (Biguer, Jeannerod, & Prablanc, 1982, 1985), and between two-handed movements (Kelso, Southard, & Goodman, 1979).

Movement may also be internally constrained by the biomechanical properties of effectors. In this case, the movement plan is assumed to be cast in terms that take into account biomechanical properties. The idea is that the movement plan specifies minimal characteristics of the movement and biomechanical properties fill in the selection from among all possible movements. For example, a desired effector endpoint might be achieved by altering the resting length (Berkenblit, Feldman, & Fucson, 1986) or the stiffness (Bizzi, 1980; Polit & Bizzi, 1978) of opposing muscle groups and then allowing the limb to spring to that position without specification of intermediate positions in the movement plan. Similarly, swinging the leg forward during walking need not involve detailed planning of the trajectory, but can be achieved by simply allowing the physical properties of the leg in a gravity field to operate (McMahon, 1984).

From the present perspective, certain difficulties arise from viewing redundant degrees of freedom and motor equivalence as a problem. First, the imposition of internal constraints to solve the problem reduces the system's ability to respond strategically to unexpected external constraints (Bullock et al., 1993). An optimized movement cannot be strategically modified online to respond to unexpected external constraints but requires offline resetting of movement parameters. Similarly, Greene (1982) argued that movements prescribed by natural synergies cannot deal strategically with unexpected external constraints without going offline. Depending on unmonitored biomechanical properties to fill in the movement trajectory amounts to assuming ballistic movements, which we argue are essentially uncontrolled and strategically unmodifiable. It seems to us that any system that imposed internal constraints to reduce freedom of movement before considering unpredictable external constraints would sacrifice the flexibility afforded by redundancy and could not evidence the hallmark of motor equivalence.

Second, although we do not minimize the computational problem posed by redundant degrees of freedom (see chapter 2), this emphasis seems somehow wrong. Stressing the problem of control posed by redundant degrees of freedom and motor equivalence obscures the strategic advantage afforded by this aspect of the motor system. Motor equivalence illustrates the flexibility of the perceptual–motor system and redundant degrees of freedom should be viewed as facilitating rather than burdening the process of perceptual–motor control (Abbs, Gracco, & Cole, 1984; Bullock et al., 1993; Saltzman, 1979).

From this alternative viewpoint, the movement plan may be conceptualized as an abstract representation that selects the set of effectors and sensors (i.e., a functional sensorimotor system) appropriate for a particular task (Buchanan, Almdale, Lewis, & Rymer, 1986; Bullock & Grossberg, 1988). This task-specific movement plan configures a subset of sensorimotor elements to cooperate toward the movement goal. Multiple actions of the linked elements are controlled in parallel and in a feedforward manner, such that perturbation in the movement of one element can be predictively compensated by adjustment in the movement of another element. Thus, redundant degrees of freedom are treated as an advantage to be strategically utilized and motor equivalence is the result of flexible response to environmental constraints. The movement plan also provides for feedback control strategically dependent on movement time and afference availability constraints. Control is, then, hierarchical, top-down from the movement plan, but also heterarchical, bottom-up from sensors (Harvey & Greer, 1980).

Such in-parallel control of compound movements utilizes internal synergistic and biomechanical constraints, but at a level below the overall movement plan, and provides for strategic response to the disturbing effects of unpredictable external constraints. How such task-specific movement plans may be acquired and how they may be translated into actual efferent commands are topics of discussion in chapter 3.

Illustrations of this kind of approach to strategic perceptual–motor performance include Abbs et al.'s (1984) model of motor programming in speech production and Bullock et al.'s (1993) neural model of reaching movements. As we show, evidence from prism adaptation supports this approach to perceptual–motor organization. In particular, the task-dependent nature of spatial realignment seems to require this kind of flexible, task-dependent specification of sensorimotor systems.

SENSORIMOTOR SYSTEMS

Our concept of a sensorimotor system corresponds to the idea of a task-dependent synergy (Buchanan et al., 1986; see also Paillard, 1991b) and to the related notion of a coordinative structure (Fowler & Turvey, 1978). However, we make explicit the role of sensors (see also, Turvey, 1990) whose function we believe to be largely involved in establishing and maintaining spatial alignment among the various parts of the total perceptual–motor system.

A minimal sensorimotor system consists of an effector, sensors, and control structures (controller) that are organized to perform a specific task. As illustrated by Fig. 1.2, we distinguish two kinds of sensors: exteroceptors, which provide information about the environment in which the controlled system operates, and proprioceptors, which provide information about the behavior of the controlled system. A controller moves the effector to achieve a performance goal specified by sensory information. Such basic sensorimotor systems can operate independently or can be coordinated by higher order planning operations.

The provision for both exteroceptive and proprioceptive functions enables autonomous behavior. Autonomy is a defining characteristic of a sensorimotor system. A sensorimotor system is a special-purpose device; an organization of sensorimotor elements to perform a specific, frequently required task, but a task that is limited in scope. The general-purpose nature of the perceptual–motor system emerges from the flexible creation and combination of such special-purpose devices (Turvey, 1990).

The strategic combination of specialized sensorimotor systems to perform more general tasks is assumed to be hierarchical in nature (see Fig. 1.2). For example, when two sensorimotor systems are combined, the nature of the linkage is such that one system assumes a controlling role and the other becomes the controlled system. We call such hierarchical combination a *guidance linkage* and assume that the linkage is directional in the sense that one system cannot simultaneously be guiding

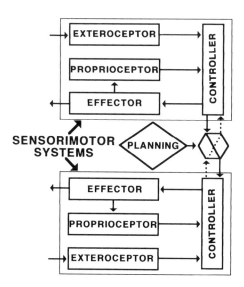

FIG. 1.2. Sensorimotor systems. A minimal, autonomous system consists of an effector, sensors (exteroceptor and proprioceptor), and control structures. Special-purpose systems can be strategically linked to produce a general-purpose perceptual–motor system.

and guided. A movement plan can, however, include nested guidance[1] linkages such that one direction of linkage can apply for part of a movement and another for a later part of the movement. Such switching in directional linkage can also be strategically sensitive to feedback. The relationship among sensorimotor systems can be described as a hierarchy–heterarchy (Harvey & Greer, 1980).

In this sense, the eye–head and hand–head are sensorimotor systems specialized for (among other things) tracking and grasping, respectively. Evidence that the eye–head is a basic sensorimotor system includes the observation that the oculomotor signal is apparently not available for visually guided limb movements. In visually guided aiming movements, visual information about the target and limb movement is expressed, not in terms of the oculomotor signal alone, but in terms of visual space (Prablanc, Echallier, Komilis, & Jeannerod, 1979; see also MacKenzie & Marteniuk, 1985). Such visual coding may reflect the organization of a basic eye–head sensorimotor system in which visual position is coded as the conjoint function of signals from the retina (exteroceptor) and extraocular muscles (proprioceptor). Such an eye–head system may be linked to a hand–head system for purposes of visually guided movements. That the guidance linkage can be reversed (i.e., proprioceptive guidance) is indicated by the fact that the eyes can track the position of the hand even when the hand cannot be seen (Gauthier, Vercher, Mussa-Ivaldi, & Marchetti, 1988).

A typical visually guided task like reaching for a coffee cup (on which the eyes have already fixated) involves a flow of control from eyes to limb. Visual information from the eye–head system is used to set the desired endpoint effector position coincident with the target. On the basis of this and the visually specified starting position of the limb, a movement plan is selected to specify the movement path. Once a movement plan has been set, the guided system enjoys a certain degree of autonomy in carrying out the plan. Proprioceptive as well as visual information may be monitored for signs of disturbance, but the use of such information is entirely local, within the hand–head system, in the sense that there is no change in direction of control from limb to eyes. Also, proprioceptive and visual feedback may be used to correct obvious errors, especially in the terminal part of the movement, but the direction of guidance is still eye-to-hand.

In contrast, looking at a wristwatch (on a stationary limb) involves the opposite direction of guidance, that is, proprioceptive guidance. Proprioceptive information from the limb must be used to select a movement plan to generate a movement path for eyes and head, which will bring the target into foveal view. The movement plan for the eye–head system is set by the hand–head system. Position sense information from both the eyes and head, as well as visual information about the movement path may be monitored for signs of disturbance, but there may be no flow of control back to the limb. Similarly, in the eye–head system, visual and proprioceptive information may be used as local feedback, without a reversal in the direction of guidance.

---

[1]This sense of the term is distinct from the guidance sometimes involved in teaching a motor skill, in which the learner is somehow guided through the task that is to be learned (Schmidt, 1988).

These examples illustrate cases where guidance may be in only one direction. Everyday skilled performance may involve several online reversals in direction of guidance, strategically deployed to maximize task performance. The skilled automobile mechanic may alternately work by sight and feel; visually guiding the hand to the general vicinity of the partially obscured nut and proprioceptively guiding the eyes and head to a better view. Even a simple movement to grasp a coffee cup usually involves proprioceptively guided eye movements to track the moving limb before it comes into view, and visual orienting toward a wristwatch usually involves visually guided limb movements to better position the wrist.

The strategic flexibility of the perceptual–motor system means that many behaviorally important sensorimotor systems are not hard wired. We argue, however, that evolutionary and physiological constraints define certain natural kinds of sensorimotor systems that constitute the basic modules of the perceptual–motor system. These basic sensorimotor systems can be strategically linked, unlinked, and relinked to flexibly perform the variety of tasks required of the perceptual–motor system. Adaptive spatial alignment is the process that assures veridical spatial communication among the components that compose a complete system.

Some of the strongest evidence for this suggested organization is the fact that under conditions of spatial misalignment, realignment occurs in the guided system (Kelso, Cook, Olson, & Epstein, 1975; Uhlarik & Canon, 1971). Direction of guidance seems to be critically involved in determining which of several spatial mappings are subject to realignment and which serve as the standard against which realignment is computed. We argue that such local realignment can occur only if the guided system includes both sensors and effectors, that is, an autonomous sensorimotor system.

FEEDFORWARD AND FEEDBACK CONTROL

Some of the basic elements of strategic perceptual–motor control were suggested almost 100 years ago by Woodworth (1899) who noted that aiming movements consist of a fast "initial impulse" phase followed by a slower "current" control phase. The terminal movement phase was assumed to be controlled by visual feedback, homing-in on the target to reduce the visual distance between limb and target. The initial movement phase can be assumed to be controlled in a feedforward manner, using predictive control to maintain the integrity of the planned movement path against disturbances. The strategic flexibility of perceptual–motor performance derives largely from trade-offs between feedforward and feedback control, each of which has its own advantages and disadvantages.

Whereas feedback control is relatively well understood, feedforward control is a confusing and confused concept. Figure 1.3 illustrates our interpretation of these two kinds of control strategies. Feedforward control utilizes the predicted sequence of the movement plan and sensed disturbances to compensate for an anticipated error before it occurs. Feedback control corrects for error after it occurs by forming an error correction based in comparison of desired and actual outcomes.

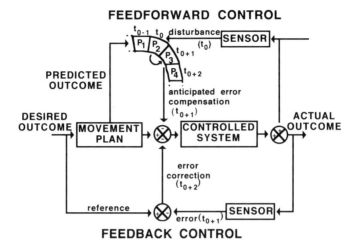

FIG. 1.3.   Feedforward and feedback control. Feedforward control utilizes the predicted sequence of
the movement plan and sensed disturbances to compensate for an anticipated error before it occurs.
Feedback control corrects for error after it occurs by forming an error correction based in comparison
of desired and actual outcomes.

Note carefully that feedforward control does *not* mean no online control (see
also Abbs et al., 1984; Abbs & Winstein, 1990; Houk & Rymer, 1981). It cannot be
the case that movements are planned and then simply released to run their course
without further monitoring. Such ballistic or open-loop movement would be
analogous to throwing one's self off a cliff. Movements with no possibility of
in-flight modification hardly would have survival value. Consistent with this view
is the conclusion from studies in electromyography (reviewed in Basmajian & De
Luca, 1985) that reciprocal inhibition of agonist–antagonist muscles in rapid
movement is affected by signals from the periphery and that "some control
algorithm other than simply presetting agonist-antagonist activation is used during
(slow) movement" (p. 228). Moreover, there is increasing behavioral evidence that
both proprioceptive information and visual information can be used to control
movement rapidly.[2]

In feedforward control, the movement plan enables a set of spatiotemporal
predictions about the sequence of joint angles that will achieve the movement goal.
When afferent information indicates a disturbance in the controlled system, say at
time t_0, potential future error can be anticipated by making an immediate compensatory adjustment in the planned sequence of joint angles, say at a later time t_{0+1}.
Because response of the controlled system to a disturbance is not instantaneous, the
feedforward controller can counteract disturbance effects before they produce an

<hr>

[2]For reviews see, Abbs et al. (1984), Abbs and Winstein (1990), Carlton (1992), MacKenzie and
Marteniuk (1985), Marteniuk (1992).

(overt) error or at least a very large error. In contrast, feedback control corrects for errors after they occur. The desired outcome is continuously compared to the actual outcome and when a deviation from the behavioral goal is detected, say at time t_{0+1}, a correction is made at some later time in the movement sequence, say at time t_{0+2}. Thus, feedforward control can produce error-free performance, at least functionally, whereas feedback control is characterized by error and error correction.

The previous definitions of feedforward and feedback control illustrate online control of submovements or from one part of a movement to the next (see also Beaubaton & Hay, 1986; Martin & Prablanc, 1992). Control may also be modified offline or between trials at a task, but here the distinction between feedforward and feedback control becomes blurred. For example, a more appropriate movement plan may be selected based on failure in a previous trial (i.e., knowledge of results[3]). Similarly, a more reliable afferent source may be monitored based on experience from previous trials. Such offline processes may be more appropriately designated as strategic parameter setting rather than direct movement control. Such offline processes may also be largely involved in more long-term development of adaptive control (discussed in chapter 3).

Probably most skilled perceptual–motor performance involves both feedforward and feedback control (Marteniuk, 1992). One often unrecognized reason feedforward control alone is not sufficient, even for highly skilled actions, is that the movement goal may be incorrectly or imprecisely specified. In such a case, the movement plan accurately predicts the movement sequence, but, if the plan is left uncorrected by feedback, the desired goal would not be achieved. Such cases include ordinary inattentive target selection and (we argue) the extraordinary case where spatial information about the target is distorted by natural processes such as growth, pathology, and normal cell death, or by artificial events such as optical distortion of visual input.

Another reason feedback control is necessary arises from the fact that feedforward control is restricted to predictable situations where a movement can be planned; a feedforward controller must have a store of schematic plans for appropriate movements in commonly occurring situations. This predictability requirement also means that feedforward control involves a knowledge of plant dynamics; a feedforward controller must have a model of the controlled system in order to anticipate its behavior. How such a store of plans and model of the controlled system might be acquired is discussed in chapter 3. The point here is that the feedforward controller may *not* have a complete plan or an adequate model. In such a case, feedback control may be necessary to fine tune the movement (Marteniuk, 1992).

There are also reasons why feedback control alone is insufficient. The principle restriction on feedback control is that afferent information must be available about the actual outcome of a movement. In an important sense, the strategic flexibility

---

[3] *Knowledge of results* seems to be a confused concept in the motor control literature. Here, we take it to mean information, in any form, about the success or failure of a movement that becomes available after completion of the movement. Thus, knowledge of results is an offline information source, in contrast to online feedback.

of feedback control is illustrated by the ability of a feedback controller to utilize a variety of afferent sources, switching to backups when one source is not available. The perceptual–motor system has proven remarkably flexible in its ability to utilize *any* available afferent information within the constraints imposed by the task (Abbs & Winstein, 1990). However, in cases where online afferent information is imprecise or completely unavailable, feedforward control based on knowledge of results may be a more effective strategy.

Another important disadvantage of feedback control is the relative slowness of such correction. Feedback correction must wait for an error to occur, in contrast to the more rapid anticipated-error compensation of feedforward control. Moreover, a closed-loop feedback control system can become unstable, propagating excessive correction around the loop in an unending cycle of oscillation (Houk & Rymer, 1981). Inclusion of an open-loop feedforward controller may guard against such instability. Also, error correction in natural systems is always incomplete and exclusive dependence on feedback control can result in a succession of smaller and smaller corrections that does not effectively null out the error before another error arises. Such failure can be minimized by employing feedforward control to arrive in the area of general accuracy and utilizing feedback control to correct for the relatively small remaining error.

Finally, the necessity for both feedforward and feedback control can be based on an argument for different evaluative functions for the two kinds of control (see also MacKenzie & Marteniuk, 1985; Schmidt, 1976). Feedforward control is concerned with maintaining the integrity of a planned movement against disturbances. Such control is more concerned with the movement plan than with the behavioral goal. The afferent sources monitored by a feedforward controller may not be directly linked to the controlled system (e.g., vision in aiming movements), but the focus is always on information about potential disturbances to the controlled system. Feedforward control is satisfied if the movement plan is achieved, regardless of behavioral goal achievement.

In contrast, feedback control is concerned that a movement achieve the particular behavioral target, for example, grasping an object. Feedback control is more concerned with the behavioral goal than with the movement plan. Again, the afferent sources monitored by a feedback controller may not directly provide information about the target (e.g., proprioception[4] in aiming movements), but the focus is always on feedback about goal proximity. Feedback control is satisfied if the behavioral goal is achieved, regardless of how the movement plan may have to be violated.

We further speculate that the information utilized by feedforward and feedback control processes may be differently coded (see also Keele, 1981, 1986; Kelso & Wallace, 1978; Schmidt & McGown, 1980). A movement plan may be couched in terms of body-relative spatial positions of the controlled effector (see also Berken-

---

[4]In the present work, we do not find it necessary to distinguish between *proprioception* and *kinesthesis* (see also Schmidt, 1988) and use *proprioception* to mean the perception of movement of body parts as well as their position in space.

blit et al., 1986; Bizzi, 1980, Bullock & Grossberg, 1988; Polit & Bizzi, 1978). Such position codes would be most useful for predictive adjustments to compensate for future disturbances in effector position. On the other hand, feedback control would be most effective if error information were coded in terms of the difference between effector endpoint and target positions (see also Bullock et al., 1993; Crossman & Goodeve, 1983; Keele, 1968; Meyer, Abrams, Kornblum, Wright, & Smith, 1988; Schmidt, Zelaznik, Hawkins, Frank, & Quinn, 1979). Such difference codes translate more directly into corrective signals to achieve the behavioral goal.

In most everyday and experimental situations, the difference between a movement plan and a behavioral goal is not distinguishable. However, the prism adaptation paradigm forces such a distinction. When the behavioral goal is erroneously encoded because of spatial distortion, a feedforward movement plan may be executed flawlessly but still not result in achievement of the behavioral goal. Moreover, feedback control may be strategically recruited to assure goal achievement, but as we see, may not address the more fundamental problem of spatial misalignment. The combination of position commands for feedforward control and difference commands for feedback control seems to be necessary for spatial realignment.

MOVEMENT SPEED–ACCURACY TRADE-OFF

The distinction between fast feedforward (predictive) control and slower feedback (reactive) control may underlie the well-known movement speed–accuracy trade-off[5] in perceptual–motor performance. Woodworth (1899) noted that in aiming movements, with a fixed time required for the movement, error at the target increases in proportion to movement distance: that is, increases in movement speed (distance/time) produce less accurate performance. Woodworth's observation was later incorporated into Fitts' Law (Fitts, 1954; Fitts & Peterson, 1964), which includes the complementary regularity that in order for an aiming movement to fall within a target of fixed width, while increasing movement distance, more time must be permitted for the movement; that is, decreases in movement speed maintains movement accuracy with increasing movement distance. This trade-off between movement speed and accuracy was verified for a variety of coordination tasks (for a review, see Keele, 1981). Some examples illustrate the large amount of empirical and theoretical work that has been directed toward movement speed–accuracy trade-off.

The Iterative-Corrections Model (Crossman & Goodeve, 1963/1983; Keele, 1968) assumes that an aiming movement consists of a series of constant duration

---

[5]We call this *movement speed–accuracy trade-off* to emphasize the operation of control processes during execution of movement and to distinguish it from the historically longer tradition of concern with the psychophysics of movement initiation (Fullerton & Cattell, 1892; Link, 1992). Although the influence of the psychophysical tradition is clear in recent models of movement speed–accuracy trade-off, we believe that the introduction of feedforward control concepts (Greene, 1969, 1972) suggests a strategic, online view of speed–accuracy tradeoff.

submovements, each taking the hand a constant proportion of the distance to center of the target and each controlled by feedback indicating the difference between current hand position and the target. Performance can be accurate by utilizing a long series of submovements, each moving the hand closer and closer to the target, but this long series of submovements will require more time for a fixed movement distance, producing overall slower movement speed. Alternatively, performance can be fast by utilizing a shorter series of submovements that requires less time for a fixed movement distance, but this short series of submovements will less accurately achieve the target. Movement speed–accuracy trade-off occurs in selecting the submovement series whose length satisfies the movement time, distance, and accuracy requirements of the task.

The Impulse-Variability Model (Schmidt et al., 1979) proposes that rapid aiming movements can be achieved in a ballistic (open-loop) manner by a neuromotor impulse timed such that the limb is forced toward the target during the first part of a movement and then coasts toward the target during the second part of the movement. Error is assumed to arise because of variability in the force driving the limb and, independently, variability in the time during which force is applied. Force variability is assumed to be proportional to the amount of force applied; time variability is assumed to be proportional to the duration of the applied force. Performance can be accurate by applying a short duration or small force, but the limb will move slowly over a specified movement distance. Alternatively, for the same movement distance, performance can be fast by applying a longer duration or larger force, but the increased variability will decrease performance accuracy. Movement speed–accuracy trade-off occurs in finding the time and force which minimizes the variability of both factors to meet task requirements (i.e., movement time, distance, and accuracy).

The Optimized Initial Impulse Model (Meyer et al., 1988) assumes a series of ballistic (open-loop) submovements of variable number (minimum of two) with each movement initiated by timed neuromotor impulses such that the relative durations and lengths of submovements are optimized to cope with variability. Variability of a submovement is assumed to increase with the distance covered by that movement and decrease with its duration; that is, error increases with increasing movement speed (distance/time). Depending on task requirements, a movement consists of a selected number of submovements. If speed is most important, one short duration, long movement enables rapid movement toward the target, but at the cost of high error at the target. Alternatively, if accuracy is most important, a series of long duration, short movements enables low error at the target, but at the cost of longer movement time for the total movement (i.e., lower overall speed for a fixed distance to the target). Movement speed–accuracy trade-off arises from finding the balance of submovement lengths and times that minimizes total movement time for a particular distance to the target (i.e., maximizes overall movement speed), within the accuracy requirements of the task.

The Vector Integration to Endpoint Model (Bullock & Grossberg, 1988) is an elaboration in the mass-spring modeling tradition (Bizzi, 1980; Feldman, 1986) in which movement is controlled by internal computation of a difference vector (DV)

between a target position command (*TPC*) and a present limb position command (*PPC*). The *DV* is assumed to change at a constant rate, but the rate of change in *PPC* increases with the magnitude of *DV.* Moreover, *DV* influences *PPC* via a multiplier whose value is set by a *GO* signal that serves to initiate or stop movement and that reflects will or arousal level.

Error at the target arises because PPC and DV may change at different rates; if PPC changes at a faster rate than DV the limb will overshoot the target before DV goes to zero and movement stops, but if PPC changes at a slower rate than DV, the limb will undershoot the target when DV goes to zero and movement stops. Movement speed–accuracy trade-off consists of adjustments of the magnitude of the *GO* signal to match task requirements (movement distance, time, and accuracy).

If the present view that feedforward and feedback control are the fundamental strategies in perceptual–motor performance is correct, then all of these accounts of movement speed–accuracy trade-off would seem to be incomplete. Perhaps the largest problem is the assumption of ballistic or open-loop movement that we believe in some sense means uncontrolled movement. Even the Iterative Corrections Model assumes that movement between feedback corrections is ballistic. Recent evidence that both proprioceptive information and visual information can be used rapidly to control movement raises the real possibility that these movements may, in fact, be under feedforward control (for reviews see Abbs et al., 1984; Abbs & Winstein, 1990; Carlton, 1992; MacKenzie & Martenuik, 1985; Marteniuk, 1992). The problem with the Vector Integration to Endpoint Model is that it involves only feedforward control, with no provision for feedback control (but see Bullock et al., 1993). The Impulse-Variability Model is similarly lacking in provision for feedback control (but see Schmidt, 1988) and the Optimized Initial Impulse Model uses feedback only to plan later ballistic submovements, not in online control.

A complete account of Fitts' Law is beyond the scope of this volume, but we do believe that a kind of movement speed–accuracy trade-off occurs in the strategic deployment of feedforward and feedback control. Speed-accuracy tradeoff may arise from the need to allow time for feedback correction of error arising from feedforward control (see also Woodworth, 1899). Feedforward control may be inaccurate because the target position is inaccurately specified, because of unexpected external constraints, because the model of the controlled system is inadequate, or because of inherent variability in the system. Such feedforward error is particularly likely when the movement distance is long or movement accuracy requirements are high (e.g., target size is small). In such cases, the feedforward movement may be slowed to allow time for feedback corrections.

Thus, a movement can be made rapidly at high speed if accuracy is less important (e.g., when distance is short and target size is large), but movement must be made more slowly at low speed if accuracy is more important (e.g., when distance is long and target size is small); a strategic trade-off between feedforward and feedback control based on requirements of the particular task. Although models that provide for both feedforward and feedback control are currently being developed (Bullock et al., 1993; Marteniuk, 1992), they have not been articulated yet to account for speed–accuracy trade-off.

Speed–accuracy considerations are obviously important for adaptive performance in the prism exposure situation. Strategic adjustment between fast-but-inac-
curate feedforward control and slow-but-accurate feedback control enables
achievement of the behavioral goal. More important for present purposes, however,
is the possibility that the speed–accuracy requirements of a perceptual–motor task
may determine whether or not spatial realignment occurs. We argue that an
exclusive emphasis on movement speed or on movement accuracy may not elicit
the kind of cooperative feedforward and feedback control necessary for spatial
realignment.

CONTROLLED AND AUTOMATIC PROCESSING

The present concepts of movement planning, feedback control, and feedforward
control may be related to the information processing concepts of *controlled processing*[6] and *automatic processing* (Schneider, Dumais, & Shiffrin, 1984; Schneider
& Shiffrin, 1977a). Schmidt (1988) summarized this distinction in the following
way: Controlled processing is "slow, attention demanding in that other similar
processes interfere with it, serial in nature, and 'volitional' in that it can be easily
stopped or avoided altogether" (p. 107). Automatic processing is "fast, not attention
demanding in that other processes will not interfere with it, parallel in nature with
various operations occurring together, and not 'volitional' in that processing is often
unavoidable" (p. 107). Of course, depending on the level of analysis, controlled
versus automatic processing is not a dichotomous distinction (Shiffrin & Dumais,
1981). At a molecular level of analysis, parts of a process may be controlled even
though other parts are automatic (Schneider & Fisk, 1983). Perceptual–motor
performance is surely such a multipart process.

Available evidence from motor control research (for reviews, see Klein, 1976;
Stelmach, 1982) suggests that controlled (attentional) processes may be required
for movement planning and initiation (Ells, 1973; Posner & Keele, 1969), for
feedback-based movement correction (Ells, 1973), and for termination of movements with high accuracy requirements (Ells, 1973; Posner & Keele, 1969; Salomi,
Sullivan, & Starkes, 1976). There is also evidence that predictable changes in
movement direction can be made automatically, but advance planning of such
direction changes is a controlled process (Klein, 1976). These conclusions have the
following implications for the present view of strategic perceptual–motor control.

The skilled actor has available a variety of movement plans appropriate for
different tasks and for different parts of an ongoing task. Choice between these
various movement plans is often a controlled process. Once a choice has been made,
maintaining the selected plan against other competing plans that are still available
may also be a controlled process. For predictable movements, the movement plan

---

[6]The meaning of *control* in this context is somewhat different from its use in the phrase *motor control.*
Controlled processing has, for example, the connotation of conscious control, in contrast to, for example,
feedforward control, which has no such intended meaning. To minimize confusion, we use *controlled*
when referring to the controlled–automatic distinction.

may be run off automatically under feedforward control at a level below the planning stage (Martin & Prablanc, 1992). When unexpected errors arise, feedback may need to be evaluated in light of the accuracy requirements of the task and a decision may be necessary about correction (see also, Proteau, 1992). Whereas execution of a correction by the controlled system may be automatic, the error evaluation required for feedback control is often a controlled process. Thus, we assume that movement planning and feedback control are largely controlled processes, whereas feedforward control is largely an automatic process. In strategic perceptual–motor performance controlled processing "is used to set and maintain the top level of a behavior hierarchy, and automatic processes execute the appropriate movements" (Schneider et al., 1984, p. 22).

Of course, the mix of controlled and automatic processing depends on the skill level of the actor. However, it seems unlikely that any task can become so highly practiced (or is so highly predictable) that only *one* movement plan is available or that accuracy requirements become completely fixed. Similarly, automatic feedforward control is unlikely always to be effective because no task is always completely predictable. Feedforward control must then, at least on occasion, be replaced by error corrective feedback control. Thus, any task for any actor is likely to involve at least some controlled processes that are subject to interference from other tasks involving similar processes. It should be noted, however, that different sensorimotor systems may not require the same controlled processes (see also McLeod, 1977, 1980) and may operate simultaneously without mutual interference. Indeed, the absence of interference is one way of identifying independent sensorimotor systems.

We argue that spatial mapping and the maintenance of alignment among spatial maps is an automatic process. This assumption is consistent with the position that sensory features are preattentively coded and spatially parallel (Treisman, 1985). Controlled, attentional processing may be required to conjoin the separate features (e.g., color, shape, motion) in a spatial region into coherent objects (see also Kahneman & Treisman, 1984; Treisman, 1992), but such object representation presumes an automatically developed spatial map in which the features are already located. The spatial alignment process is activated by perceptual–motor processes that link spatial maps so that misalignment can be detected, but the fact that these perceptual–motor processes (e.g., planning and feedback control) may often be controlled processes does not change the automatic nature of spatial alignment. It does suggest, however, that spatial alignment cannot be investigated without careful scrutiny of the strategic perceptual–motor processes required by the experimental task.

SUMMARY

The picture we have painted is of a highly flexible perceptual–motor system. Its repertoire includes a store of special-purpose autonomous sensorimotor systems, possible organizations of effectors, sensors, and control structures that can be strategically recruited and linked and relinked in the variety of ways that gives the total perceptual–motor system the character of a general-purpose device. Online control of movement consists of a strategic mix of feedforward and feedback control to meet the speed–accuracy requirements of the task. Movement planning and feedback evaluation are commonly controlled processes, but feedforward control and movement execution are largely automatic processes. Adaptive spatial alignment is an automatic process that maintains spatial communication among the various sensorimotor systems, but activation of spatial alignment depends on strategic perceptual–motor control processes that link misaligned sensorimotor systems. In chapter 2, we consider the nature of the spatial medium of communication among sensorimotor systems.

Chapter 2

SENSORIMOTOR TRANSFORMATION

It is a truism "to say that any description of a given state of matter is frame dependent" (Paillard, 1991a, p. 471). Such spatial frameworks are fundamental to our perceptual and motor experiences. Different spatial frameworks underlie perception and motor mechanics, and perceptual–motor integration can be thought of as transformation among reference frames (Simpson & Graf, 1985). In this chapter we first examine the various kinds of reference frames that can be identified for the perceptual–motor system. Then we consider how information in particular frames of reference may be represented (coordinate systems or maps) to define structured spaces. Finally, we discuss the nature of the rules governing transformations among the various perceptual–motor spaces and note some suggested transformational mechanisms.

More specifically, we develop the hypothesis that perceptual–motor representation is a hierarchy–heterarchy (see Harvey & Greer, 1980) of three-dimensional coordinate spaces. Position in each space is described by three degrees of freedom for location (left–right, near–far, up–down) and three degrees of freedom for orientation (pitch, roll, yaw), with separable representations for location and orientation. The various spaces are related by homeomorphic (topological) and unique, direct and inverse transformations of translation and rotation. Spatial alignment between origins and axes of the various coordinate systems is achieved by parametric adjustment in these transformations. Adaptation to common prismatic displacement and tilt, then, can be viewed as a parametric change in transformations of translation and rotation, respectively.

REFERENCE FRAMES

Perceptual–motor theory employs a variety of descriptive spatial systems, variously called *spaces* (Saltzman, 1979), *coordinates* (Soechting, 1989), and *maps* (Jeannerod, 1991b). All of these terms carry certain implications about geometric structure. A more structurally neutral term is *frame of reference* (Paillard, 1991a; Simpson & Graf, 1985). A *frame of reference* is a set of lines or planes used to describe spatial position. The notion of a reference frame implies some "space," some set of points endowed with a structure, usually defined by a set of axioms to be satisfied by the points. We defer consideration of geometric structure until the next section. The following typology of reference frames (summarized in Fig. 2.1) is meant to be neutral with respect to a particular structure.

Environmental frames describe spatial location and orientation in the task–work space of the organism. Two kinds of environmental frames are commonly distinguished (Paillard, 1991a): *body frames* describe the task–work space in terms centered on the body; *object frames* describe the task–work space in terms centered on objects. Environmental frames are extrinsic in the sense that a particular frame may be chosen more or less arbitrarily for convenience of description with little regard for the intrinsic nature of the perceptual–motor system. Nevertheless, extrinsic frames provide the objective foil for inferring the nature of intrinsic frames and are themselves modified with changing conceptualization of intrinsic frames. For example, the distinction between body and object frames both suggests and is suggested by the distinction between the sensorimotor mode (knowing where) and the representational mode (knowing what) of information processing (Paillard,

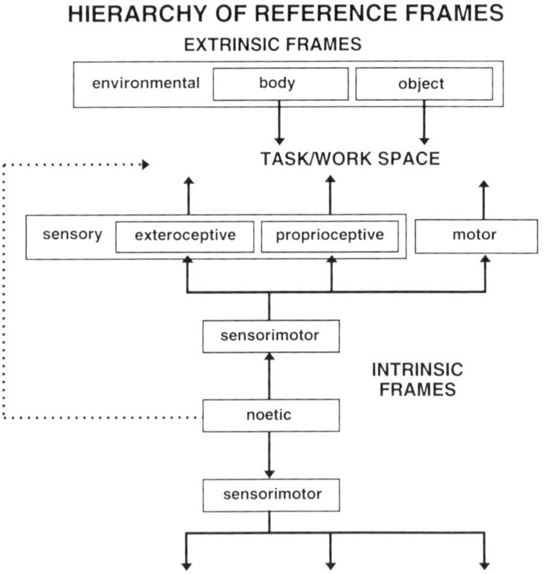

FIG. 2.1. Hierarchy of reference frames. Extrinsic Environmental frames provide objective body-centered and object-centered descriptions of the task–work space. Intrinsic (kinematic) Sensory frames and (dynamic) Motor frames describe regions of the task–work space, centered on exteroceptors, proprioceptors, and effectors. Intrinsic Sensorimotor frames describe the region of task–work space for a sensorimotor system (i.e., exteroceptor, proprioceptor, and effector). Noetic frames provide intrinsic descriptions for combined sensorimotor frames that closely approximate the entire task–work space as described by extrinsic frames.

1991a, 1991b) and subserving neural organizations (Mishkin, 1993; Ungerleider & Mishkin, 1982).

Sensory frames describe a region in which perceptual measurement of the task–work space of the organism can take place. Two kinds of sensory frames may be distinguished (Jeannerod, 1992; Jeannerod & Biguer, 1982; Soechting, 1989): *proprioceptive frames* describe a region of personal space, the portion of the task–work space within the boundary layer (e.g., the skin) of the organism; *exteroceptive frames* describe a region of extrapersonal space, the portion of the task–work space beyond the boundary layer. Sensory frames are *intrinsic* (natural) in the sense that a particular description is suggested by the organization of the biological system. For example, the sensory frame for global spatial analysis may be defined by the principle axes of the semicircular canals of our ears or body planes (Simpson & Graf, 1985).

Motor frames describe changes in effector position (i.e., movement) within a region of the task–work space of the organism. Two intrinsic levels of motor frames must be distinguished (Simpson & Graf, 1985; Soechting, 1989): *kinematic frames* describe movements without reference to the forces that produce them, and *dynamic frames* describe movements in terms of forces. Dynamic frames are obviously required to describe muscle action. Kinematic frames are also necessary because perceptual processes describe pure movement, although kinematics may specify dynamics (Kelso & Kay, 1987). Kinematic frames may, then, be thought of as sensory frames and, with this classification, motor frames are exclusively dynamic in nature.

Sensorimotor frames are regional descriptions of the task–work space defined by the organization of sensory and motor frames into specialized sensorimotor systems. Prototypical examples of such specialized sensorimotor systems include the mouth, the eyes, and the hand (Paillard, 1991b; see also, Grobstein, 1988, and Sparks, 1988). In the case of a sensorimotor system, personal and extrapersonal space is not a dichotomous distinction because mobile effectors and associated proprioceptors describe regions of the task–work space beyond the boundary layer.

The overlap of personal and extrapersonal space is defined by the range of action (reach) of the effector (i.e., the kinematic frame). When a sensorimotor system includes an exteroceptor the boundary of the sensorimotor frame is further extended to the perimeter of the exteroceptive frame. Moreover, the usual differential articulation among regions of an exteroceptive frame arising from narrowly focused exteroceptors (e.g., vision and touch) is corrected by integration within a sensorimotor frame. That is, as the effector moves the exteroceptor around, the current portion of the sensorimotor frame is specified by the proprioceptor. Thus, sensorimotor frames map personal space (proprioceptive frames) onto extrapersonal space (exteroceptive frames) and enable perceptual–motor behavior throughout an expanded region of task–work space.

To this basic catalog of reference frames we would make one addition. Sensorimotor frames are centered on the particular collection of effectors and sensors that define a sensorimotor system. Hierarchical linkage of sensorimotor systems creates a reference frame that is centered on the collection of subsystems. The collection of all sensorimotor systems, or any subset that spans the body trunk, defines an intrinsic description that at least approximates the extrinsic body frame (Abend, Bizzi, & Morasso, 1982; Flash & Hogan, 1985; Morasso, 1981; Shepard, 1981; see also Soechting, 1989). A body-centered description that emerges from the organization of sensorimotor systems we call a *noetic frame*.[1] By specifying an egocentric description of the task–work space, a noetic frame of reference provides a common means of communication among the various parts of the perceptual–motor system, no matter how the various sensorimotor systems are organized into subgroupings to perform particular tasks.

As an illustration, the retina, extraocular muscles, and eye position sensors contribute exteroceptive, motor (kinematic), and proprioceptive frames, respectively, which combine to create a head-centered, eye–head sensorimotor frame. Similarly, the tactile receptors, muscles, and position sensors of the lower limb contribute exteroceptive, motor (kinematic), and proprioceptive frames, respectively, which combine to create a limb-centered, hand–arm sensorimotor frame. Sensorimotor organization to perform, for example, visually guided limb movements, involves reorganizing the extension of subsystems to include mediating articulations (e.g., eye–neck and hand–shoulder) to create a trunk-centered, noetic frame of reference. A noetic frame defined by a different sensorimotor organization is still a body centric description. For example, the linkage of ear–neck and hand–shoulder systems to silence the morning alarm clock involves a noetic frame centered on the body. In this manner, the perceptual–motor system has a description of the entire task–work space potentially available.

SPACES, COORDINATES, AND MAPS

The assignment of geometric structure to a reference frame specifies a particular space. Environmental space is, as we presently understand it, locally Euclidean and three-dimensional (3-D; Paillard, 1991a; Shepard, 1989), as illustrated in Fig. 2.2. The 3-D structure of egocentric body space (Howard, 1982) is specified by a gravitationally conferred unique upright dimension (Z) corresponding to the vertical midbody axis (up–down), a second dimension (Y) that is orthogonal to both gravity and the midsagittal body plane at the body's center of gravity (left–right), and a third dimension (X) in the midsagittal plane orthogonal to the other dimensions at the center of gravity (near–far).

Assignment of a metric to the set of dimensions enables description in terms of a coordinate system. Egocentric location is specified by distance coordinates along these body axes and egocentric orientation is specified by angular rotation about

---

[1]The idea a noetic frame might be extended to correspond with an allocentric representation of the body in relation to the environment, a geocentric world frame (e.g., Paillard, 1991a, 1991b), but such an extension seems unnecessary for present purposes. In any case, this kind of representation is assumed to be built up from exteroceptor and proprioceptor input, not directly given by hypothetical "exteroproprioceptors" (e.g., Lee, 1980).

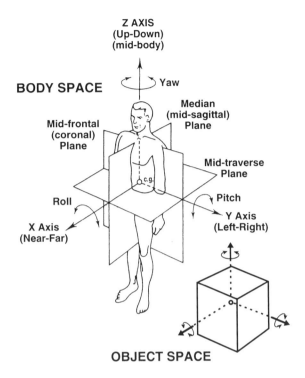

FIG. 2.2. Coordinate system for position in body space and object space. Location is specified in coordinates along independent axes of 3-D Euclidean space and orientation is given by angular rotation about the axes. The origin of coordinate axes for body space is the center of gravity (c.g.). Adapted from *Human Visual Orientation* (p. 6), by I. P. Howard, 1982, New York: Wiley. Copyright 1982 by John Wiley and Sons. Adapted with permission.

the Z-axis (yaw), the Y-axis (pitch), and the X-axis (roll). Motion is described in terms of translation along and rotation about these coordinate axes (Shepard, 1984; Simpson & Graf, 1985). Object space is similarly specified in three dimensions, but with the coordinate system centered on an object.

A clarifying distinction can be made between the number of spatial dimensions and the number of coordinates (and coordinate systems) required for complete spatial specification in an n-dimensional space. For example, complete specification of spatial position in 3-D Euclidean space requires six coordinates (degrees of freedom); three for location and three for orientation. The number of coordinates is sometimes called the *dimensionality* of the spatial representation. This higher dimensionality, however, arises from the need to represent multiple spatial attributes (location and orientation) in 3-D space (Shepard, 1989). Location and orientation may be thought of as represented by separate 3-D coordinate systems with distance and angular metrics, respectively.

It is reasonable to assume that the 3-D Euclidean nature of the terrestrial environment imposes natural spatial constraints that have shaped our body architecture during the course of evolution. These natural constraints have produced intrinsic spatial representations that have a geometric structure similar to the (at least locally) 3-D Euclidean world (Paillard, 1991a; Shepard, 1989). For example, the separable nature of location and orientation in environmental space is paralleled by separable neural systems for sensorimotor and object representation (Mishkin, 1993; Paillard, 1991b). This natural separation is also reflected in distinct sensorimotor systems for control of endpoint location for the limb and grasping orientation of the hand (Jeannerod, 1992, 1994; Jeannerod & Biguer, 1982; see also Georgopoulos, 1986, 1990). However, intrinsic spatial representation may also be constrained by the physical nature of the representing system.

Obvious constraints on intrinsic representation of 3-D space are the two-dimensional (2-D) nature of receptor surfaces and the underlying neural medium. For exteroceptive senses like vision and touch, the 3-D world is available only in the reduced form of its projection onto a 2-D sensory array. This 2-D projection is preserved in topographic mappings onto layers or sheets of neural tissue that are also essentially 2-D in structure. Both receptors and the central nervous system would seem, therefore, to be incapable of representing depth.

However, the missing dimension can be recovered by representing depth nontopographically as the magnitude of neural activity in different regions of the topographic map (Shepard, 1989). And, depth itself can be computed from depth indicators available in the patterned input. Even with nontopographic coding of depth, exteroceptive space can only represent the 3-D world from a particular, momentary vantage point. However, when an exteroceptor is mobilized by an attached effector and with proprioceptive input, exteroceptive space can be extended to create a general 3-D sensorimotor space with coordinates centered on the sensorimotor system.[2]

Intrinsic representation of (kinematic) proprioceptive space is constrained by mechanical limits on movement. For example, upper limb position can be represented with two coordinates of location and one of orientation, position of the lower limb segment requires one coordinate for location and one for orientation, and hand position can be described by two coordinates of location (see Fig. 1.1).[3] Complete specification of arm position requires seven coordinates, but this description is built up from intrinsically constrained 3-D coordinate systems for each limb segment.

---

[2]Fundamental topology tells us that "the relations between objects in a space of three dimensions cannot all be preserved in a two-dimensional projection. . . . It is ultimately the variability and incompleteness of the view afforded us by our dimensionally reduced window on the world that leave us irremediably susceptible to occasional perceptual solecism and deceptions" (Shepard, 1990, pp. 173–175). However, our representation of the world is remarkably good for most purposes.

[3]Limb location coordinates are usually expressed as the relative angle formed between limb segments at their common joint (for a review, see Soechting, 1989). Such angle coordinates, however, assume a fixed length for limb segments; an assumption that is surely not valid during early development. The point coordinates in 3-D space for the distal end of a limb segment is, therefore, probably the more intrinsic form of limb representation.

The natural origin for each local coordinate system is the proximal joint for each limb segment. When one segment is linked with another to form a special purpose sensorimotor system, the superordinate coordinate system (sensorimotor space) is centered on the more proximal point of articulation.

The high dimensionality of proprioceptive limb space arises from the many degrees of freedom required to specify location and orientation for each body segment in 3-D space. It may be, however, that each limb segment is represented separately in the neural medium[4] by, at most, three coordinates (Georgopoulos, 1990). The in parallel, hierarchical–heterarchical control of the limb described in chapter 1, therefore, need specify, at most, only three coordinates for each limb segment. Coordination of the separate segments could be achieved automatically by the carryover of position of a more proximal segment to the origin of the coordinate system of a more distal segment. A movement plan could be specified by the required position of each limb segment in a sensorimotor limb space (Soechting, 1989) and commands sent simultaneously to each segment, with coordination achieved by the natural hierarchical linkage among separate coordinate systems for the limb segments.

Another example of constraints on proprioceptive space is the mechanical limit on translational movement of the eye along the axes of 3-D space. Only small translations are possible and an adequate description of the eye in the head may be given in terms of rotation alone (Simpson & Graf, 1985). Thus, a kinematic description of eye position and movement requires only three coordinates of rotation about the axes of 3-D space centered on a notional point fixed by both the eye and the orbit. When linked to the trunk via the neck, the origin of the eye-in-head coordinate system (proprioceptive space) is shifted by changes in head position (location and orientation), defining a region of personal (noetic) space centered on the body.

Thus far, we have seen how the assumptions of hierarchical levels of representation, separable representations for location (translation) and orientation (rotation), and mechanical constraints on movement of body segments may limit the dimensionality of spatial representations to no more than three (and perhaps fewer) coordinates. At the level of intrinsic (dynamic) motor space matters would appear to be more complex. For example, the six eye muscles each define an axis of force capable of rotating the eye (Robinson, 1975; Simpson & Graf, 1985). The dimensionality of eye motor space would seem to be six, one coordinate for the state of each eye muscle. However, by averaging agonist–antagonist muscle pairs, three notional muscle rotation axes can be created (Ezure & Graf, 1984a, 1984b; Robinson, 1982, 1985). In this manner, three coordinates might be sufficient to specify an eye position, one for the relative activation levels for each pair of eye muscles. Similarly, motor spaces of relatively low dimensionality might be defined for limb segments in terms of agonist–antagonist muscle synergies. Thus, the structure of (dynamic) motor space may match the associated (kinematic) proprioceptive space in dimensionality.

---

[4]As previously noted, the 2-D neural medium may be augmented to three dimensions by the local magnitude of neural activity.

In this section we show how the various intrinsic reference frames (exteroceptive, proprioceptive, motor, sensorimotor, and noetic) may be assumed to have a 3-D Euclidean structure. Moreover, we argue that in an hierarchically organized perceptual–motor system, with separate representations for spatial location and orientation, the dimensionality of a spatial representation need not be greater than three coordinates, and, with mechanical constraints on effectors, even fewer coordinates may be required. Having specified the geometric structure of the various spaces (exteroceptive, proprioceptive, motor, sensorimotor, and noetic), we now turn to a consideration of how information is heterarchically exchanged among these spaces to enable perceptual–motor behavior.

TRANSFORMATIONS

Our discussion of intrinsic spatial structure suggests that, at least at higher levels of perceptual–motor interaction, communication among the various sensory and motor spaces is mediated, in part, by relatively simple translation and rotation transformations of coordinates from one coordinate system to another. These are natural transformations in our 3-D Euclidean world and are likely to have been embodied by evolution in our body architecture at all levels of organization.

For example, egocentric position for a visual target can be represented by first coding target location and orientation (perhaps separately) in 3-D, retinocentric (exteroceptive) space. Target position in eye–head (sensorimotor) space can then be determined by applying translation and rotation transformations to retinocentric coordinates; the magnitude of rotation being given by eye position in the head (i.e., proprioceptive space). That is, retinocentric coordinates are adjusted for the known separation between origins of retinocentric and head-centric spaces (translation) and for present eye position (rotation). Egocentric direction available in proprioceptive space augments egocentric depth available in exteroceptive space to specify an extended, but head-centric, sensorimotor space.

The reverse linkage to fixate an alternate target could be achieved by applying inverse transformations that specify the eye rotation needed to bring the fovea to the target in retinocentric space. That is, given a separation between targets, the required change in egocentric direction (and depth) can be computed in sensorimotor space and transferred as a rotation to eye muscles (motor space), adjusted for (translation) the known separation between origins of exteroceptive and proprioceptive spaces. Eye movement would be sensed in (kinematic) proprioceptive space and direct transformations[5] would provide the basis for monitoring the movement in sensorimotor (eye–head) space.

For multijoint systems like the hand–shoulder illustrated in Fig. 2.3, the account

---

[5]We use the terms *direct* and *inverse transformations* to refer to sensory input and motor output processes, respectively. This usage contrasts with the terminology of mechanics (e.g., Simpson & Graf, 1985), where direct transformation refers to the case where components of a movement are known and the task is to determine the resultant movement, and inverse transformation is the case of determining the components of a known movement.

is complicated only by the number of transformational steps required. For example, hand position in hand–shoulder (sensorimotor) space could be determined by first coding hand position in 3-D wrist-centric space, then applying translational and rotational transformations to transform coordinates into elbow-centric and shoulder-centric space. We assume that multiple transformations occur in parallel, such that hand position can be changed by applying inverse transformations that specify interdependent (synergistic) positions for limb segments (see chapter 1).

Linkage of sensorimotor systems would require further transformations into noetic space. For example, linkage of eye–head and hand–shoulder systems would require additional rotation and translation to take into account present head position and provide a common reference in terms of body-centric space.

Of course, motor commands would also have to be transformed from kinematic (movement path) representation into dynamic (muscle force and torque) representation. A similar, but inverse transformation from dynamic to kinematic representation would also have to be performed to make available sensory information (i.e., proprioceptive space). The requirement of transformation between kinematic and dynamic representations does not, however, change the underlying nature of the transformations.

Note carefully that we assume spatial representation for a body segment to be 3-D even when freedom of movement may be lower in dimensionality. For

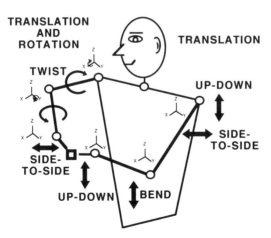

FIG. 2.3.   Transformations among limb segment coordinate systems. Coordinates axes are shown for each limb segment, centered on the immediately proximal joint. With up–down, side-to-side, and bending movements of the arm, coordinate axes for the three segments are related simply by translations (left arm of figure). With twisting movements, coordinate axes are related by both rotations and translations (right arm of the figure).

example, the lower limb has only two degrees of freedom; one for location (bending at the elbow) and one for orientation (rotation about the segment's longitudinal axis). Moreover, the range of movement is limited in each of these dimensions. Nevertheless, we assume the basic structure of spatial representation to be 3-D throughout the perceptual–motor system for three reasons.

First, as previously argued, the basic 3-D structure of environmental space can be assumed to have dictated the evolution in structure of intrinsic spatial representation.

Second, and perhaps most convincing, limb positions that are mechanically impossible can, nonetheless, be perceived when effector movement is prevented but continued changes in muscle afference are induced by artificial means (Craske, 1977; Goodwin, McCloskey, & Matthews, 1972; McCloskey, 1973; Skavenski, Haddad, & Steinman, 1972). Mechanical limitations are, then, only mechanical limitations, not limitations on spatial representation.

Third, and most convenient, by assuming an invariant 3-D structure and separate spatial representation for location and orientation, we avoid the complicating problem of overcompleteness in spatial transformation (Llinás & Pellionesz, 1985; Simpson & Graf, 1985). When the dimensionality of one reference frame is greater than another, transformation from the first frame to the second is said to be indeterminate (overdetermined, overcomplete, or nonunique) because the transformation yields not just one solution, but an infinity of solutions. The inverse of such a transformation may be unique, but because transformation must be done in both directions (e.g., sensory-to-motor and motor-to-sensory), differences in dimensionality among spatial representations poses a formidable computational problem (Jordan & Rosenbaum, 1989; Saltzman, 1979).

It should be noted, however, that if the present simplifying assumptions about spatial representation ultimately prove untenable, available computational procedures for overcomplete transformations (Llinás & Pellionisz, 1985; Pellionisz, 1984, 1985; Pellionisz & Llinás, 1985; see also Churchland, 1986) may be incorporated into the present view without violating the more fundamental idea that rotation and translation are basic transformations in perceptual–motor processing. Moreover, the nature of the transformations that map one space onto another and the kind of computational mechanism(s) that will solve the overcompleteness problem may be separable issues. For the present, then, this perhaps oversimplified view of spatial representation enables us to specify in a relatively straightforward manner the problem of spatial alignment, which we see as the central problem addressed by prism adaptation research.

SPATIAL ALIGNMENT

We distinguish between processes that translate and rotate coordinates between coordinate systems and processes that set equation parameters for translation and rotation. That is, transformation of coordinates requires parameters that compensate for sets of axes that may not be parallel and whose origins do not coincide. Such parameters normally have long-term, steady-state values and translation or rotation of coordinates is commonly automatic and transparent (Shepard, 1981) in everyday perceptual–motor coordination. However, these parameters are not permanently fixed. For example, the translation required by length of the upper limb between shoulder-centered and elbow-centered coordinate systems is usually fixed by adulthood, but changes drastically during early development. Similarly, differences in orientation among the optic axes, the principle axes of the semicircular canals, and body planes (Simpson & Graf, 1985) require rotation parameters that are relatively constant during adult life but that may require adjustments over the course of development.

We are now able more exactly to define what we mean by adaptive spatial alignment. *Spatial alignment* is the application of fixed-value transformation parameters to compensate for long term, steady-state differences in origin location and axes orientation between coordinate systems. *Adaptive spatial alignment* is the necessary adjustment in parameter values to maintain alignment of coordinate systems.

Normal sources of change in alignment (misalignment) are slow acting, requiring small parameter changes; for example, slow drift arising from normal cell death and growth. Misalignment, however, may be large and sudden, as in pathology with massive cell loss and experimental distortion of sensory input (e.g., prism adaptation). The prism adaptation paradigm has unique advantages for the study of adaptive spatial alignment because the magnitude and onset of misalignment is known.

This view of prism adaptation was first suggested to us by Dodwell's early essay (1970) in cognitive science. Dodwell noted that conformal[6] translation and rotation closely approximate the commonly studied optical displacement and tilt of the visual field, respectively. He suggested that adaptation might consist in finding the inverse of the transformation to remove the distortion. We now believe that translation and rotation (and their inverses) are natural transformations that mediate exchange of information among the various spatial representations of the perceptual–motor system. Prismatic distortion activates processes of parameter adjustment in transformations that normally serve to maintain alignment among the several spatial representations.

The simplest conformal transformation is translation. For the simple case of two dimensional spaces ω and z, the translation of z onto ω is given by $\omega = z + A + Bi$, where A and B are real numbers specifying translation along the two axes. When optical displacement changes the existing alignment between origins of the two spatial coordinate systems, adaptation may consist in finding the new value for parameters A or B or both that will reestablish mapping between corresponding

---

[6]Conformal transformations are a subset of isogonal transformations that preserve sense of rotation as well as equiangular intersection. A conformal transformation between two-dimensional planes, mapping points in z onto ω, is expressed by the relation $\omega = F(z)$, where z is the complex number, $x + iy$, expressing a vector with the two independent coordinate values. The inverse, $F^{-1}(\omega) = z$, maps points in ω onto z. Conformal mappings that are biuniform (homeomorphic), such that one-to-one mapping holds in both directions, provide close approximations for most prismatic distortions (Dodwell, 1970).

points in the two spaces. We assume that knowing the new parameter value(s) for one direction of mapping also enables the inverse transform for veridical mapping in the opposite direction. In subsequent chapters, we are concerned with how this basic process of spatial alignment fits into the larger process of perceptual–motor coordination. As such, we do not attempt to provide precise mathematical descriptions of the transformations. Dodwell's observations, however, point to a direction in which a more quantitative statement might be developed.

Another early influence on our thinking was the observation that, although adaptation to prismatic displacement and tilt of the visual field is parametrically similar in magnitude, growth, and decay functions (Redding, 1973b, 1975a), the perceptual–motor system can adapt as well to simultaneously imposed displacement and tilt as to each distortion separately (Redding, 1973a, 1975b). Thus, adaptation to displacement and tilt appeared to be served by similar, but separable mechanisms.

We now believe that these two kinds of adaptation involve similar kinds of spatial alignment parameter adjustment (for translation and rotation transformation, respectively) but in separable representations for location and orientation. We suspect that such separable representations are related to distinct neural systems for sensorimotor and object representation. How these two neural systems interact is currently a topic of intense research in cognitive neuroscience (e.g., Jeannerod, 1992, 1994; Mishkin, 1993; Paillard, 1991a) and we hope that the present account of prism adaptation may contribute to understanding the associations and dissociations between these two systems.

A confirmation of our approach to adaptive spatial alignment is the observation that visuomotor adaptation to translation of visual space (Bedford, 1989) and rotation of motor space (Cunningham, 1989) generalizes more or less completely to all spatial positions, showing little or no gradient around training positions (see also Paillard, 1991b).[7] At least for these transformations (but see Bedford, 1993a, 1993b), mapping between visual and motor spaces involves connecting entire dimensions, not a collection of individual visual–motor associations. In terms of the present formulation, such rigid shifts in spatial mapping functions occur because natural translation and rotation specifies the alignment between spatial coordinate systems and an artificially induced parameter change in a transformation alters the correspondence relationship between all points represented in the different spatial coordinate systems. Separate computations for each position are not necessary; a general relationship is established (see also Bedford, 1993a). Any and all positions

---

[7]Bedford's (1989) finding that a rigid shift occurs between training points (interpolation), but not necessarily beyond training points (extrapolation) might be explained in terms of the present hierarchical framework. If exposure training restricted realignment to the spatial relationship between more distal, subordinate limb spaces (e.g., wrist to lower limb), but postexposure testing required positioning in a more proximal, superordinate space (e.g., limb to shoulder), then the reduced range of the training space would appear as absent extrapolation in the larger test space. Consistent with this explanation is the fact that locus of realignment with Bedford's experimental paradigm is largely in limb space rather than in the larger range of visual space (Bedford, 1993a). However, Bedford (1993b) offered other theoretically motivated accounts for the absence of extrapolation that also may have to be considered.

in one coordinate system are automatically, transparently transformed into corresponding positions in another coordinate system.

SUMMARY

We argue that perceptual–motor representation is a hierarchy–heterarchy of 3-D coordinate spaces and perceptual–motor integration can be thought of as transformations among the various spatial representations. The various spaces are related, in large part, by homeomorphic and unique, direct and inverse transformations of translation and rotation, which reflect the natural structure of our locally Euclidean 3-D world. Transformations are normally automatic and transparent, enabled by parameters that compensate for coordinate systems whose axes may not be parallel and whose origins do not coincide. Such spatial alignment may, however, be altered by growth, normal drift, pathology, or distortion of sensory input. Adaptation to misalignments produced by prismatic displacement and tilt can be viewed as parameter changes in transformations of translation and rotation, respectively. Adaptive spatial alignment, however, is only one kind of learning that can occur in the prism adaptation paradigm. In chapter 3, we consider the varieties of learning.

Chapter 3

PERCEPTUAL–MOTOR LEARNING

Having sketched the perceptual–motor organization that enables strategic (task-dependent) perceptual–motor control (chapter 1) and the representational basis of perceptual–motor control (chapter 2), in this chapter we turn to the question of learning—how the structural and representational bases of perceptual–motor control are acquired.

First, we elaborate on Bedford's (1993b) functional classification of types of learning, adding a contrast between specialized and general acquisition processes. In this context, we characterize adaptive spatial alignment as a kind of specialized (domain-specific) knowledge acquisition process for learning (veridical) matches among internal sensory and motor spatial representations.

Next, we examine various instances of perceptual learning. We suggest that perceptual learning includes one general acquisition process (differentiation) and a variety of specialized acquisition processes, including adaptive spatial alignment.

Then, we examine data and theory from motor learning (skill acquisition). We conclude that adaptive motor control is a kind of general (associative) knowledge acquisition process for matching one's internal states to those of another, different in kind from adaptive spatial alignment.

Finally, we outline how an organization around sensorimotor systems may offer a unique solution to the problem of achieving correspondence between the structure of intrinsic and extrinsic space given only the constraints available from intrinsic representation.

VARIETIES OF LEARNING

There are many different kinds of learning. More than half a century's intensive research demonstrates most clearly that learning is not some monolithic entity. But categorization of kinds of learning is made especially difficult by the proliferation of learning types that occurred during the last 10 years, spurred by interest in modules (Fodor, 1983) and domain-specific acquisition systems (Rozin & Schull, 1988). Such proliferation requires some classification scheme to organize the varieties of learning. Bedford's (1993b) functional classification is a tentative scheme that is particularly useful for present purposes.

The top portion of Fig. 3.1 reflects Bedford's (1993b) classification of experiences that make us better in terms of three kinds of learning: world learning, perceptual learning, and other learning. The bottom portion of Fig. 3.1 is an additional classification in terms of restrictions on what can and cannot be learning: specialized (domain-specific) and general acquisition processes. We first sketch Bedford's classification and then overlay the distinction between specialized and general acquisition.

Bedford began by identifying learning with effects of experiences that make us better, in contrast with effects of experience like fatigue and injury that make use

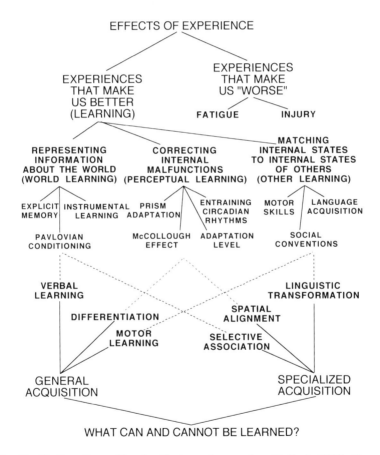

FIG. 3.1.   Classification of types of learning. The top portion reproduces Bedford's (1993b, Figure 1) functional classification in terms of what is learned. The bottom portion (below dashed lines) shows an additional distinction in terms of specialized acquisition that is largely constrained by genetic endowment and general acquisition characterizing more arbitrary learning. From "Perceptual Learning," by F. Bedford, 1993b. In D. Medin (Ed.), *Psychology of Learning and Motivation*, 30, p. 3. Copyright 1993 by Academic Press. Reprinted with permission.

worse (see also Lorenz, 1981; Rozin & Schull, 1988). Learning is most often regarded as a process that enables us to apprehend the new information about the world available from experience, represented in Fig. 3.1 by the associative processes in Pavlovian conditioning, instrumental learning, and (explicit) memory. Such *world learning* involves acquiring an internal knowledge representation of the world, "matching one's own internal states to the world" (Bedford, 1993b, p. 4). Other kinds of learning, however, can be distinguished.

Perception provides information about the momentary state of the world, but perception is too important and complex to be learned from scratch by each individual organism "through trial and possibly fatal error" (Shepard, 1984, p. 432). The more fundamental regularities (structures) of our world (e.g., its locally Euclidean nature) are stable enough to have been embodied in the genetic makeup of organisms (see also Biederman, 1987, 1990; Spelke, 1990; Spelke, Breinlinger, Macomber, & Jacobson, 1992). In an important sense, individuals already know the most predictable aspects of the world. This knowledge is embodied in perceptual mechanisms.

World learning consists of apprehending the less predictable aspects of the world, available through the normally transparent operation of perceptual mechanisms. The primary function (adaptive value) of perceptual learning is to ensure that perceptual information sources are operating optimally.

These perceptual mechanisms, however, operate differently in different stimulation contexts and are prone to specific, infrequent but predictable malfunctions. *Perceptual learning*, from this view, is the adaptive capacity to correct for expected malfunctions of these genetically given perceptual mechanisms and to adjust their operation in contextually appropriate ways. Bedford suggested that a perceptual malfunction is often, if not always, indicated by discrepancy between representations produced by different perceptual mechanisms. Perceptual learning usually involves "matching one's own internal states to one another" (Bedford, 1993b, p. 4).

As examples of perceptual learning, Bedford offers (a) *prism adaptation,* which reflects the adaptive capacity to maintain veridical intermodality spatial mapping in the face of (for example) physical growth; (b) the *McCollough effect,* which reflects the adaptive capacity to filter out orientation contingent color fringes (see also Bedford & Reinke, 1993; Held, 1980); (c) *adaptation level,* which reflects the adaptive capacity to maintain maximal sensitivity to differences in sensory magnitudes when average sensory magnitude changes; and (d) *entraining circadian rhythms,* which reflects the adaptive capacity to maintain an accurate internal clock with changes in onset of light and dark periods. These examples suggest that perceptual learning might, perhaps more properly, be characterized as *plasticity*—changes in the operation of perceptual mechanisms that seem to be learning and not learning at the same time.

Bedford (1993b) suggested a third and somewhat special category (i.e., *other learning*[1]) for learning in a social context that consists of acquiring internal knowledge representations that correspond to internal knowledge representations

---

[1]Bedford does not so name this category, but we suggest *other learning* as an appropriate name.

of other people, "matching one's own internal states to the internal states of others" (p. 4). In this case, what is learned is not so much external states of the world or one's own internal states as it is the structured internal states of other people. For example, language acquisition consists of matching your language to someone else's language, social conventions are acquired to match your rules of proper behavior with someone else's rules, and motor skill usually involves acquiring what someone else can do. Such representations also account for the ability to perceive the intentions of other people.[2]

In later sections of this chapter we discuss the validity and implications of placing perceptual learning and motor learning (skill acquisition) in separate categories, distinct from world learning. First, however, we attempt to draw out another way of distinguishing among different kinds of learning. Implicit in Bedford's classification is the idea that evolution and learning differentially contribute to different kinds of knowledge (see also Rozin & Schull, 1988). The bottom part of Fig. 3.1 illustrates this idea in terms of what can and cannot be learned because of evolution's contribution.

Specialized acquisition processes are constrained by evolution to operate in more restricted domains and can only learn more specific kinds of knowledge from experience. For example, the McCollough effect may represent specialized acquisition of the contingent relationship between retinal image orientation and the color fringes produced by the ocular prism (Bedford & Reinke, 1993; Held 1980). *General acquisition* processes are less constrained by evolution and can learn more arbitrary kinds of knowledge from experience. For example, instrumental learning (operant behavior) illustrates general acquisition of a wide variety of more or less arbitrary relationships between stimuli and correct (reinforced) responses (behavior). Note that general acquisition should not be confused with the frequency or distribution of a process in the human system. For example, adaptation level is a ubiquitous process, but specialized for each application. General acquisition is, in the extreme, arbitrary in what can be learned.

A brief consideration of the structure of knowledge provides a somewhat crude but heuristic way of talking about what learning is required for a particular kind of knowledge. If we can think of knowledge as some established relationship(s) among some set(s) of elements, then evolution and learning can be thought to differentially contribute to specifying the set(s) of elements to be related or the relationship(s) or both. The more stable (predictable) aspects of the environment are likely to already be "known." It is the more arbitrary (variable) aspects that must be learned. Perhaps the most variable aspect of a knowledge structure and most likely to be learned is its elements. Relationships are more stable across a variety of elements and more likely to be genetically recorded.

We believe it is not entirely a consequence of emphasis that Bedford's examples of perceptual learning tend to be specific "devices," whereas examples of the other kinds of learning tend to be general processes. Specialized acquisition processes

---

[2] For a discussion of this point, see Jeannerod (1994).

are simply more common in perception. The most stable relationships in our environment long since have been wired into our perceptual mechanisms, and the experience of an individual largely contributes only in learning the various elements that can enter into the relationship. Moreover, perceptual learning is limited to the kinds of relationships internalized by evolution.

For example, we argued (chapter 2) along with Bedford (1993a) that intermodality spatial mapping (especially, spatial alignment) is governed by a limited class of functions, with a few modifiable parameters (see also Hay, 1974). The form of a function reflects an evolutionarily internalized representation of a particular aspect of the locally Euclidean space in which the organism has evolved. The organism is limited in the spatial mappings that can be learned to this class of genetically given functions, and perceptual learning consists largely in changing parameter values. In contrast, higher cognitive knowledge is much less constrained by evolution and more arbitrary elements and relationships among elements can be learned (see also Bedford, 1993b; Koh & Meyer, 1991). Traditional verbal learning is a tour de force in arbitrary elements and relationships. We argue that motor learning, at least at its more abstract levels, must also be such a general acquisition process in order to afford the various arbitrary and exotic skills that can be learned.

Specialized acquisition is not, however, restricted to perceptual learning. For example, language acquisition likely involves experience-based selection of the linguistic transformations specific to a particular language from among the genetically permissible transformations characterizing all human languages (for a review see Stillings et al., 1987). Specialized acquisition in world learning may be illustrated by selective association (e.g., conditioned taste aversion) in which the set of elements that can be related, if not the relationship itself (for a review see Rozin & Schull, 1988), is genetically determined. Also, perceptual learning may not be without general acquisition processes. Differentiation (Gibson, 1969, 1984) may be a general perceptual process whose function is to enable the organism to "pick up" on (learn) the task relevancy ("affordance") of information (especially higher order structure) that the perceptual system has evolved to provide.

The variety of learning, then, arises both from the different functions served and from the degree of specialization in content. Different kinds of learning can be distinguished that serve to represent new information about the world, to correct the operation of perceptual mechanisms that provide information about the world, and to acquire skills that other people have. In each of these functions, however, the acquired content may be characterized as a specialized *plasticity* or general *learning,* depending on how much of the knowledge structure is stable (in evolutionary time) and has been genetically recorded.

PERCEPTUAL LEARNING

With the exception of E.J. Gibson's differentiation process described in the previous section, there are almost no general theories of perceptual learning. Rather, one usually finds listings of specific instances of perceptual learning (Epstein, 1967;

Hall, 1991). We take this as some evidence that perceptual learning exists largely in specialized acquisition devices rather than general processes. Specialized plasticity is characteristic of perceptual learning because specific mechanisms have evolved to record certain remarkably stable features of our world. We call the operation of these mechanisms, or the result of applying this kind of knowledge, *perception*. Perceptual learning exists largely in specialized adaptive capacities to make adjustments in specific perceptual mechanisms.

Perhaps the most extensive catalog of candidate types of perceptual learning was provided by Epstein (1967). Epstein distinguished five classes in terms of the types of studies that investigated perceptual learning. In this section, we discuss these classes in relation to the classification system just discussed and to the present concern with adaptive spatial alignment.

The first class of studies investigating the effects of *long-established, extraexperimental past experience* would probably not now be considered instances of perceptual learning. These studies of, for example, size–distance and shape–slant relationships in perception (see also Epstein & Park, 1963; Epstein, Park, & Casey, 1961) are probably best seen as illustrations of the effects of evolutionary endowment (Shepard, 1984). Experimental manipulations of the "assumptive context" can be seen as selecting a particular genetically given internalized world regularity, rather than learning. If there is perceptual learning involved in these kinds of studies, it is perhaps of the differentiation type; learning to discriminate the internalized regularities (perceptual mechanism or information source) that are relevant to particular tasks. Note that although an internalized regularity may be in terms of higher order variables, it may also be accessed in terms of first order variables. We see no reason to assume that the elements of a relationship are lost in the representation of the relationship (cf. Gibson, 1950, 1966; see also Shepard, 1984).

The second class of studies investigating the effects of *controlled experimental training or practice* includes a variety of enrichment, transfer of training, verbal labeling, reinforcement, and goal-directed behavior manipulations (see also Hall, 1991). We believe that most, if not all, of these kinds of studies can be viewed as motor learning. *Motor learning,* we shortly argue, consists of the general acquisition of largely arbitrary associative linkages between differentiated input–output states. Again, the only kind of perceptual learning that may be involved in such studies is differentiation.

Epstein's third class of *cue-conflict* studies (Wallach, Moore, & Davidson, 1963) and his fourth class of *prism adaptation* studies (Kohler, 1951/1964) may be grouped together as instances of specialized acquisition devices for matching internal states—that is, perceptual learning in Bedford's sense. The model of adaptive spatial alignment we develop in chapter 6, however, elaborates on Bedford's matching of internal sensory states to add matching between sensory input states and motor output states. It is not enough to correct for any intrinsic misrepresentation of extrinsic space; if an organism is to do anything with its knowledge, it is also necessary to assure that intrinsic space maps back onto extrinsic motor space. We believe that adaptive spatial alignment and most, if not all, of the cases included in Epstein's third and fourth classes involve learning internal matches among both sensory and motor states.

Epstein's final class, *developmental studies,* is largely beyond the present scope. We would only note that the various specialized acquisition devices for calibrating internal states are surely active in perceptual development. Moreover, the general acquisition process of differentiation is arguably the basis for much perceptual development (Gibson, 1984). We do not, however, uncritically assume that perceptual development in the child is the same as perceptual learning in the adult.

Insofar as we can see, then, perceptual learning consists of perhaps one general acquisition process (differentiation) for learning the task relevancy of the perceptual information sources (mechanisms) that evolution has provided and a variety of specialized acquisition devices for maintaining the calibration of the so-provided internal representations. Moreover, because such calibration must surely also involve output motor states, it is not clear that there is ever pure perceptual (input) learning. Even differentiation is seen as providing the basis for learning motor output organization (Gibson, 1984). In the following section we examine whether motor learning of input–output relationships might not be a better way of conceptualizing such learning.

MOTOR LEARNING

In this section we present an associative view of motor learning in which the learned goal behavior is isomorphic with the hierarchical control structure outlined in chapter 1. *Motor learning* is the acquisition, through practice and, more generally, experience, of skilled movements that are maximally efficient and goal-directed (Schmidt, 1988).[3] The to-be-learned goal behavior is usually specified by other people who already have the requisite motor skill. Motor learning consists of organizing a control structure that enables the learner-actor to match the behavior of other skilled performers. Because people are (presumably) structurally similar, similar control structures underlie similar skills, and learning a motor skill consists in "matching internal states to internal states of others" (Bedford, 1993b, p. 4). Thus, *skill acquisition* can be viewed as the construction of an internal representation that captures the neural and physical, as well as behavioral aspects of the goal behavior.

The top portion of Fig. 3.2 illustrates a possible structure of the goal behavior representation and the course of skill acquisition. The to-be-learned goal behavior is a set of associative linkages between particular sensory input patterns (from exteroceptors and proprioceptors) and particular motor output commands (to effectors), spatially and temporally organized to enable skilled performance. Learning the goal behavior (i.e., goal-directed learning; Marteniuk, 1992) is a matter of selectively discriminating the relevant input and output, so they can be contiguously associated. In this view, motor learning is a kind of directional associative learning

---

[3]Motor learning is distinguished from maturation of genetically given components of perceptual–motor control, although such components are prerequisites of skilled performance.

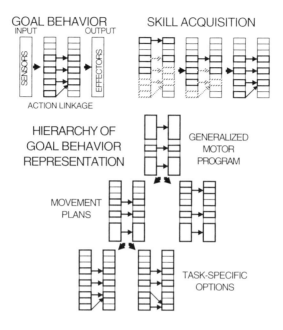

FIG. 3.2.   Skill acquisition. The to-be-learned goal behavior is described as action linkages between differentiated input–output elements and skill acquisition is characterized as an increasingly specific (accurate) internal representation of the goal behavior. Different hierarchical levels of a goal behavior representation include the abstract Generalized Motor Program, increasingly specific Movement Plans, and various task-specific options.

in which the input–output association is an action linkage similar, at least, to a production rule (Anderson, 1983, 1987; Masson, 1990/1991). The course of skill acquisition can be largely described as increasing differentiation of the inputs and outputs required for the goal behavior; that is, increasing specificity (accuracy) of input–output content for the internal representation of the goal behavior.

A traditional characteristic of skill acquisition is the development of "automaticity," by which the skill can be performed without awareness and without interference from other information processing activities (Fitts, 1964; James, 1890; Pew, 1966). The development of automaticity can be explained by increasing specificity of associative linkages (Proteau, 1992; Schmidt, 1987). Early in skill acquisition, the input–output contents required for the goal behavior are only coarsely known. At this stage, interference from other information processing activities is large because input–output may include extraneous content that is also involved in other information processing activities and conscious attentional selection is largely involved in trying out various sensory sources of information and motor organizations. As skill at the task develops, input–output content becomes more specific to the task and overlaps with the content of fewer other information processing activities. Moreover, increasing specificity means that skilled performance can be unconsciously triggered by an increasingly circumscribed set of circumstances; that is, there are fewer or no choices about the input–output relationship. Thus, the course of skill acquisition can be characterized as a progression from controlled toward automatic processing (Schneider & Shiffrin, 1977b; Shiffrin & Schneider, 1977).

Specificity of learning (Henry, 1968) can also explain the relative effectiveness of active, response-produced feedback (Schmidt, 1987) and more cognitive information sources like observation (Adams, 1990/1991), mental practice (Feltz & Landers, 1983), and augmented feedback (Newell, 1976). The goal behavior may be grossly identified by simply observing other people who have the desired skill, but simple observation is rarely, if ever, sufficient to identify the subtleties of input and output required for skilled performance. Like observational learning, mental practice can identify some of the more salient content of a skill, particularly on the input side, but it cannot provide the finer details, especially about output organization. For example, imagined movement can provide only limited information about biomechanical properties of effectors. Because the information provided is more focused on the particular task, augmented feedback can substantially facilitate skill acquisition, but the verbal nature of such information means that it cannot completely inform the actor-learner about the goal behavior. Ultimately, practice at the task and response-produced feedback is required to complete differentiation of the input–output content of the goal behavior.

Moreover, specificity of learning can account for the goal-directed nature of changes in feedback control over the course of skill acquisition (Proteau, 1992). A more accurate (specific) representation of the goal behavior enables improvement in error detection and feedback control (Schmidt, 1987), because both the desired output is more clearly defined and the most informative input is identified. Error correction facilitates associative learning (Adams, 1971; Schmidt, 1975) by changing input–output content to more closely match the goal behavior. Error correction selects, for associative linkage, more accurate input patterns and more successful output organizations.

Motor learning, then, requires learning to selectively discriminate (differentiate) the specific sensory variables (Gibson, 1969, 1984; Schmidt, 1987), and the specific motor organization (Proteau, 1992; Young & Schmidt, 1990) required for the skill and the course of skill acquisition consists of increasing specificity of input–output content (Masson, 1991; Marteniuk, 1992; Proteau, 1992). Such discrimination learning delivers an increasingly more accurate representation of input–output contents of the goal behavior, which can then be associatively linked by contiguous "pairing." In this respect, motor learning is similar to stimulus and response learning in the traditional paired-associate paradigm of verbal learning (e.g., Kausler, 1974), although motor learning often involves learning to discriminate higher-order variables (Fitts, Bahrick, Noble, & Briggs, 1961; Fuchs, 1962; Gibson, 1969, 1984).

A specificity of learning view cannot, however, account for generalization across variable instances of a task and transfer of skill components to similar tasks. In the extreme, generalization and its measured effect, transfer, must be considered learning *failures*—failures to discriminate the particular input–output contents of the goal behavior. Although generalization and transfer are limited (Marteniuk, 1992; Proteau, 1992), they are undeniably part of motor learning (Schmidt, 1988).

The bottom portion of Fig. 3.2 illustrates how generalization and transfer are accommodated by assuming a hierarchy of goal behavior representation (Greene, 1972; Schmidt, 1988). Because input–output contents are represented at varying levels of abstraction, associative linkages at higher levels of the hierarchy constitute general plans for a variety of similar tasks, with the more specific input–output contents (parameters; Schmidt, 1975) for a particular task being given at lower levels of the hierarchy. Hierarchical skill learning is still based in contiguous pairing of differentiated input–output contents, but more or less simultaneously at all levels of the hierarchy. Generalization or transfer occurs because the associated input–output contents describe general classes (categories) of goal behaviors. Moreover, the set of particular input–output contents grouped under a superordinate movement plan represent the various means (strategies) for achieving a particular behavioral goal (i.e., motor equivalence described in chapter 1).

The highest level in the hierarchy of goal behavior representation corresponds to the generalized motor program (Jordan, 1990) or schema (Schmidt, 1975). As originally conceived (Keele, 1968; Schmidt, 1975), acquisition of a program or schema, with its embedded connections to lower levels in the hierarchy, was thought to enable a change from closed-loop (feedback) control to open-loop control where error feedback is not required for skilled performance. After all, the hallmark of skill acquisition is the reduction, even disappearance of errors. More recently (Abbs et al., 1984; Jordan, 1990; Marteniuk, 1992), however, skill acquisition has been recognized as involving a change from feedback control toward feedforward control (see chapter 1).

In skill acquisition a feedforward controller is learned that "knows" the characteristics of its extrinsic task–work space; both the controlled system (e.g., biomechanical properties of the effector plant) and any external system with which it may be interacting, such as a tool. With this knowledge, impending errors can be detected by monitoring early disturbances of input and can be corrected (online) before they occur, or become very large. Error correction is the occasion for associative learning of feedforward motor programs. The consistent occurrence of an error producing output with an earlier disturbance signal and contingent pairing of the input with the corrected output enables the formation of predictive linkages, such that occurrence of the disturbance signal activates the corrective output before the error occurs. It is probably necessary to assume that some learning of feedforward control schemes occurs at all levels of the hierarchy of goal behavior representation, but the greatest amount of generalization or transfer is afforded at the most abstract level.

Figure 3.3 summarizes this view of motor learning, showing how it relates to the control structures illustrated in Fig. 1.3. Unlike the simplification in Fig. 1.3, the Movement Plan in Fig. 3.3 does not directly provide a control signal, because, as we hope to show, it is not separable from the feedforward controller but is part of the hierarchically organized control structure. We make no claim of presenting a new model of motor learning. Rather, this figure presents the consensus we see in motor learning theory in a way that most clearly shows the associative and hierarchical nature of motor learning.

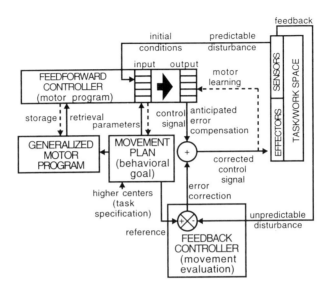

FIG. 3.3.   Motor control and learning. Skill acquisition consists of learning a (predictive) feedforward controller at different levels of the hierarchical control structure. Learning a feedforward controller is implemented by feedback error correction to differentiate the desired output and sensory consequences to differentiate the desired input, so that input–output can be contiguously associated to establish an action linkage.

In learning, higher, goal-setting centers initially specify the behavioral goal in terms of its general input characteristics (sensory consequences). Along with initial conditions from the task–work space, the behavioral goal is loaded onto the input side of the input–output associative interface. This initial input configuration selects, by associative linkage, an initial output (control signal) whose sensory consequences approximate the behavioral goal. The selection is based in previous learning of similar tasks or in genetically given linkages. In this sense, learning is never completely from "scratch." The resulting movement is evaluated (feedback controller) by comparison of the sensory consequences of the control signal applied to effectors with the consequences specified by the behavioral goal (reference).[4] The feedback controller provides a difference between desired (reference) and actual (feedback) outcomes that is used to correct the control signal to effectors (error correction). Thus, the feedback controller assures that learning is goal directed (see also Kawato, Furukawa, & Suzuki, 1987).

---

[4]The output control signal from the feedforward controller that produces movement and the reference to the feedback controller that evaluates movement are analogous in function to Adams' (1971) memory trace and perceptual trace and to Schmidt's (1975) recall memory and recognition memory, respectively.

Error correction provides the basis for adaptive change in the associative interface on both the input and output sides. The corrected control signal is used directly to modify output content of the interface, providing a control signal that avoids the error. This process is labeled *motor learning* in Fig. 3.3, but motor learning also involves contingent change of input content. Predictable sensory consequences of the corrected action modify input content of the interface, such that the conditions resulting from the corrected control signal are added to the conditions that produced the error.[5] Repeated trials serve to both increasingly differentiate relevant input–output contents when errors occur and strengthen the associative linkage at the interface even when errors do not occur. In this manner, initial conditions and predicted errors become associated with a control signal that compensates for the error before it occurs.

Slow movements during learning are necessary to build up the linkages that enable predictive control during an extended, complex movement. However, even rapid movements during learning can establish linkages that can anticipate those errors that are predictable from the task–work space conditions existing before a movement begins. That is, for simple movements the requisite control structure may be entirely specified by premovement conditions and the feedforward controller may be learned with rapid movements where feedback is available only after the movement has been completed.

Learning a feedforward controller involves simultaneously learning input–output contingencies at different hierarchical levels. At a more abstract level is learned an input–output inverse of the predictable output–input relationships in task–work space, that is, a sensory-to-motor inverse of the motor-to-sensory transformation. This learned mapping relating control signals (output) and movement outcomes (input) represents a schematic knowledge of task–work space predictability, limited only by the sampling imposed during training. These boundary conditions can be expanded by training with different tasks, but in the same work space. Such an abstract schema constitutes a generalized motor program that can be recruited for a variety of activities in the same task–work space. The subordinate set of predictable input–output relationships specific to a particular task is learned at a lower level. Such a specific movement plan for achieving a behavioral goal constitutes the parameters imposed on a generalized motor program to realize goal-directed control for a specific task. Note carefully that the labels *Generalized Motor Program* and *Movement Plan* in Fig. 3.3 are intended to designate different levels of organization of the feedforward controller. They are not memories separate from the control structure.

---

[5]In effect, the feedforward controller is learning both to predict control signals from their sensory consequences (an inverse model of the task–work space) and to predict the sensory consequences of control signals (a forward model of the task–work space). In the case in which the controlled system is nonlinear and the relationship between control signals and sensory consequences is many-to-one (overcomplete), the forward model could be used to select one "correct" control signal (Jordan, 1990; see also Jordan & Rosenbaum, 1989). We suggest a more intuitive account of how the degrees of freedom problem is solved.

The movement plan is itself learned with increasing specificity at lower levels in the hierarchical control structure (see Fig. 3.2). At higher levels, a movement plan includes the general configuration of sensorimotor systems to be recruited for the task and articulation of the goal behavior is in terms that can benefit from more cognitive information sources like observation, mental practice, and augmented feedback. At lower levels, kinematic and dynamic details of the movement are determined, for which active, response-produced feedback is needed.

Thus, the various ways in which a task might be performed (i.e., degrees of freedom) at an abstract level of representation are reduced to a single, specific task configuration at the lowest levels of representation. Moreover, experience with task variations enables the feedforward controller to acquire alternative "branches" (task-specific options) and the ability to strategically vary the selected control structure depending on particular task conditions (i.e., motor equivalence). Note also that the variety in kinds of sensory information among different levels of the control structure enables the feedback controller to be strategically sensitive to whatever kind of feedback information may be available.

We assume that a learned control structure is accessed (retrieved) at levels of the goal-directed movement plan. The generalized motor program does not include a goal specification but can be used to facilitate learning another goal-directed behavior for the same work space (i.e., showing transfer). Because we believe purposeless behavior, if it occurs at all, is rare, we assume that the generalized motor program is usually inaccessible. The more abstract levels of a movement plan can be retrieved with abstract (e.g., verbal) information about the task–work space and behavioral goal. However, if task variants have been learned at lower levels of the control structure, strategic changes in performance will appear as the relevant performance-based sensory information needed to select among the several subordinate control structures becomes available. To the extent that predictable input–output relationships have been learned at all levels, an activated feedforward controller can compensate for an error anticipated from a predictable sensory disturbance, showing near error-free performance.

For the rare case of closed skills (Poulton, 1957), in which input–output relationships are perfectly predictable, learning a feedforward controller can become complete (i.e., showing error-free performance) by between-trials' feedback adjustments to the control signal if the required movement is simple. For complex movements, learning a closed skill can be completed by momentarily slowing the movement so that the corrected output can be associated with its input conditions; that is, feedback control is employed to "fine tune" the imperfect feedforward controller (Marteniuk, 1992). In the more common case of open skills, in which input–output relationships are not perfectly predictable, a perfect feedforward controller cannot be learned. Movement must either be slowed to permit online feedback correction, or some amount of error must be accepted as tolerable (Proteau, 1992). We assume that movement speed and acceptable error level are general task specifications, strategically set by higher decision centers (see chapter 1).

Clearly, motor learning theory is richly articulated, in contrast to perceptual learning theory. It is also clear that some perceptual (input) learning, as well as motor (output) learning, is involved in skill acquisition, if only in terms of the general acquisition process of differentiation. Although motor learning theory generally has not directly addressed the problem of spatial alignment (see Bullock et al., 1993), the learned sensorimotor transformations necessary for skill acquisition may also offer an account of adaptive spatial alignment. We examine this possibility in the next section.

ADAPTIVE SPATIAL ALIGNMENT

Recall from chapter 2 that *adaptive spatial alignment* is defined as adjustment in the parameters of specialized transformations that align origin locations and axis orientations of coordinate systems for various intrinsic spatial representations. Adaptive spatial alignment is, then, an instance in Bedford's (1993b) class of matching internal states. However, we are reluctant to characterize this kind of learning as *perceptual* because we recognize the necessity of including intrinsic motor representations as well as intrinsic sensory representations. As we suggested in chapter 2 and develop more fully in chapter 6, we believe that communication between sensory and motor space is mediated by noetic space, and transformation from noetic to motor space is the inverse of the direct transformation from sensory to noetic space. Thus, a change in "perceptual" parameters entails a change in "action" parameters and we feel justified in claiming that adaptive spatial alignment is truly *perceptual–motor learning*.

A principle difficulty we see with current motor learning theory is the absence of any provision for noetic representation. Exclusively concerned as it is with producing an action that has the desired sensory consequences, the motor-to-sensory (perceptual) transformation is entirely attributed to characteristics of the task–work space (muscle plant and any external system) and the learned control structure provides the inverse, sensory-to-motor (action) transformation. In short, there is no provision for perception and no clear recognition that sensory signals have their own unique characteristics that must be transformed before they are intelligible to effectors. Simply associating arbitrary inputs and outputs will not do. They must be expressed in the same "language" for action plans to be developed. Still, there is some indication that motor learning theory is on the way to correcting this deficiency. For example, Jordan's (1990) "forward" model of the task–work space is a learned motor-to-sensory transformation and might be used to enable perception.

Another problem is that, as currently conceived, motor learning is a general acquisition process. Such a general knowledge acquisition process is necessary to account for the large variety of arbitrary and even exotic skills that can be learned. Motor learning, therefore, contrasts with the specialized knowledge acquisition that seems to characterize adaptive spatial alignment. This limitation is mitigated by the assumption of more specialized devices at increasingly lower levels of the learned control structure (Bullock & Grossberg, 1989; Bullock et al., 1993), and specialized adaptive capacity at less abstract levels of the control structure might be able to accommodate spatial alignment (Gaudiano & Grossberg, 1991).

However, another related and even more fundamental problem is the seeming commitment to the *General Process Theory* of learning (Rozin & Schull, 1988) that holds that learning is composed of a few basic, associative processes that are the same across all domains. This commitment seems especially clear in recent neural network theories of motor learning (Gaudiano & Grossberg, 1991; Jordan, 1990). Such exclusively associative theories predict that competence will be limited to that region of the domain sampled in training (i.e., the traditional generalization gradient) and cannot account for the complete competence across the domain with limited sampling that seems to characterize adaptive spatial alignment (Bedford, 1989, 1993a, 1993b; see also Paillard, 1991b). Adaptive spatial alignment involves learning parameter changes for a genetically given transformation, not learning the transformation itself, and such learned parameters apply across the entire domain of the transformation. Note that the fact that an associative network can learn a similar transformation (Gaudiano & Grossberg, 1991) may only mean that such a system can learn *anything* (see also Shepard, 1989), not that associative learning is the basis for adaptive spatial alignment. To the extent that current motor learning theory is committed to General Process Theory, it would seem unable to explain adaptive spatial alignment.

Whether current motor learning theory can be extended to explain adaptive spatial alignment depends on elaboration of the perceptual side of motor control, identifying the corresponding low-level specialized control structures, and demonstrating that associative learning principles can produce parameter adjustment for fixed transformation rules. The model we develop in chapter 6 is, we believe, nonassociative, and, although adaptive spatial alignment is fitted in and dependent on motor control structures, we do not believe that motor learning is directly involved in the process. Now, in the last section of this chapter, we consider a problem that is fundamental for either an associative or a nonassociative view of adaptive spatial alignment.

CORRESPONDENCE PROBLEM

Given that one important kind of learning involves acquiring and maintaining veridical matches among intrinsic spatial representations, there are certain logical difficulties in achieving this kind of learning. Namely, the transformation(s) among intrinsic spaces must be such as to preserve their correspondence with extrinsic space, but this cannot be achieved directly because extrinsic space is not known except as given by intrinsic representations. We call this the *correspondence problem*: How is the correspondence between the structure of intrinsic and extrinsic spaces achieved given only the constraints available from intrinsic representation? Its solution involves several steps and alternatives.

A necessary first step is to determine when a difference between spatial representations signals an error in representation and not something out in the world.

Only after an internal error (discordance) has been detected can correction (adaptation) occur. One approach is to assume that the intrinsic representations are of the same object (Bedford, 1993b; Radeau, 1994). Then, any difference between representations must be due to error because evolution has endowed the knowledge that for the same object to have different spatial attributes is an impossible state of the world. But how can the *object–unity assumption* (Welch & Warren, 1980, 1986) itself be justified and under what conditions is one object assumed instead of more than one object? One justification appeals to cross-modal application of Gestalt principles (Radeau, 1994) viewed as knowledge of world regularities endowed by evolution.[6]

The principle of *proximity* (i.e., spatial contiguity) reflects the world regularity that spatially similar stimulation is more likely to come from the same object than from different objects. So, small differences in spatial attributes (e.g., size, location, orientation) between object representations in different intrinsic spaces are more likely to evoke assumed object unity (and identification of an internal error) than are large differences. The principle of *common fate* (i.e., temporal contiguity) reflects the world regularity that temporally synchronous stimulation is more likely to come from the same object than from different objects. So, small asynchronies between object representations in different intrinsic spaces are more likely to evoke assumed object unity (and identification of an internal error) than are large differences.

This appeal to Gestalt principles almost seems circular (see also Bedford, 1994): Differences that are not regarded as differences are regarded as errors! Moreover, it raises the problem of specifying a (presumably low) threshold difference beyond which object unity would not be assumed, and internal error would not be corrected (cf. Radeau, 1994). Perhaps most critically, correcting errors in intrinsic spatial representation is localized at a high level in perceptual processing, after object representations have been formed (Biederman, 1990), that seems inappropriate for such a vital process as adaptive spatial alignment. Also, it raises Held's paradox (Bedford, 1994): Is object unity necessary for internal error correction or does internal error correction enable object unity?

Another solution to the problem of discriminating internal errors from world states is possible if we assume active, exploratory, sensorimotor systems rather than passive, receptive, perceptual systems. The intrinsic organization of the perceptual–motor system is such that synchronous actions of sensorimotor systems are usually initiated by the same target in extrinsic space. For example, eye–hand coordination is, by definition, initiated by a single extrinsic position. The *common action* (coordination) principle reflects the intrinsic regularity that synchronous actions are more likely to be directed toward the same target than different targets. After ordinary performance error has been accounted for, any remaining difference between the involved spatial representations can be identified as internal error (cf. Gaudiano & Grossberg, 1991). Common action does not require object-level process-

---

[6] For other instances where Gestalt principles are interpreted as internalized regularities of the world (i.e., constraints) see Biederman (1990) and Marr (1982).

ing but only target spatial structures (e.g., location and orientation) that may be available before or separate from object representation. Thus, common action justifies a target unity assumption and provides for object unity after internal error correction (see also Bedford, 1994).[7] The efficacy of common action, however, depends on being able to separate internal error from ordinary performance error. In chapter 6, we show how this can be achieved using feedback to correct ordinary performance error and feedforward (corollary discharge) signals to detect internal error.

Another overlooked aspect of the correspondence problem is that internal error cannot be detected by directly comparing modality-specific spatial representations. Visual and proprioceptive spaces, for example, are fundamentally incommensurable. That is why transformations are necessary! A flawed transformation cannot be detected by using the flawed transformation. There are additional arguments to be made for the necessity of some kind of noetic representation (see chapters 2 and 6), but certainly one reason is that noetic space provides the common "metric" by which internal error can be detected. Generally, an internal error is indicated when transformations from modality-specific (or sensorimotor) spaces do not pick out the same spatial structure in noetic space.

Detection in noetic space of an internal error does not, however, indicate the source of the error. Remember, that although noetic space is good approximation of extrinsic space, it is built from sensorimotor spaces. There is no direct access to the environment. A detected internal error could arise from any or all of the sensorimotor spaces compared in noetic space. The problem is to determine where to make the correction. Which transformation's parameters should be adjusted? There is no quick fix for this problem. We believe that an interim solution is achieved by adjusting the parameters of the spatial representation for the guided sensorimotor system into agreement with those of the guiding sensorimotor system. The "worker" believes what the "boss" tells him. The variety of interchange of "boss" and "worker" roles required by everyday perceptual–motor coordination assures that the total system and its various parts will ultimately settle on veridical representations of extrinsic space. Craske (1975) suggested a similar account of veridical cross-calibration of spatial representations.

The solution to the correspondence problem we outlined here constitutes a substantial part of our model of adaptive spatial alignment (chapter 6) and accounts for much of the data from prism adaptation research (chapters 4 and 7). Other aspects of the model implied by this sketch include the organization around sensorimotor rather than perceptual systems (cf. Bedford, 1993b; Radeau, 1994), a view of nonassociative dimensional learning (Bedford, 1993a) rather than associative pairwise learning (cf. Jordan, 1990), and online internal error correction

---

[7]Object unity is not, however, entirely dependent on having corrected internal error. The literature on intersensory interactions (e.g., Radeau, 1994; Welch & Warren, 1980, 1986) suggests that object unity can be assumed, with consequential dominance relationships among discrepant sensory attributes, but without correction of the internal error (see also Welch et al., 1979). In chapter 7, we show how such cross-modal integrations can occur in our proposed perceptual–motor structure and how they may actually limit internal error correction (see also Welch, 1994).

enabled by feedback–feedforward discrimination of error source rather than an offline "babbling" phase to isolate internal error correction (viz., system identification) from other error sources (cf. Bullock et al., 1993).

SUMMARY

In this chapter, we argued that prism adaptation (especially adaptive spatial alignment) involves learning matches among internal states, distinct from learning matches between internal and world states (world learning) or learning matches between internal states and the internal states of others (other learning). Furthermore, this kind of learning includes matching motor states and should be characterized as perceptual–motor learning (sensorimotor systems) rather than perceptual learning (perceptual systems). Moreover, such learning is an instance of specialized (domain-specific) knowledge acquisition, rather than the general knowledge acquisition characteristic of motor learning. Finally, organization around sensorimotor systems suggests common action as a means of establishing (veridical) correspondence between spatial structure in intrinsic representations and extrinsic space. Next, in chapter 4, we examine the features of the research paradigm for prism adaptation that make it uniquely suited to investigation of learning matches among internal states and list some of the principal results from this paradigm that suggest the model of adaptive spatial alignment developed in chapter 6.

PART II

PRISM ADAPTATION

Part I distinguished among strategic perceptual–motor control (chapter 1), adaptive spatial alignment (chapter 2), and the distinctive kinds of learning involved in these two components of adaptive perceptual–motor performance (chapter 3). With this background, we now turn to consider, in Part II, how these adaptive processes are evoked by the prism adaptation paradigm.

In chapter 4, Paradigm and Generalizations, we sketch some history and outline the distinguishing methodological features of the prism adaptation paradigm. In this chapter, we draw several generalizations from prism adaptation research that constrained the model of adaptive performance developed in chapters 5 and 6.

In chapter 5, Contributions of Strategic Control, we first develop a model of strategic perceptual–motor organization and then show how such a system responds adaptively to the performance problem posed by the prism adaptation paradigm. The specific adaptive processes that we suggest are feedback compensation, feedforward (knowledge-of-results) compensation, and associative learning. We conclude chapter 5 with the observation that, although strategic control can produce adaptive performance, it cannot solve the more fundamental problem of spatial misalignment.

Chapter 6, Alignment and Realignment, extends the model of perceptual–motor organization to include processes for adaptive spatial alignment. We distinguish among alignment (transformations for spatial mapping among sensorimotor frames), calibration (expression of the present spatial relationship among sensorimotor elements), and realignment (parametric change in spatial mapping functions). This chapter, we believe, constitutes our most unique contribution to adaptive perceptual–motor performance.

Chapter 7, Theoretical Issues, discusses traditional issues in prism adaptation in the context provided by the theoretical framework of the preceding two chapters. First, we identify the multiple adaptive processes (postural adjustment, strategic control, and realignment) evoked by the prism adaptation situation. Then, we show how known conditions for realignment (reafference, performance error, and selective attention) can be understood in the present framework. We conclude this chapter with a discussion of how the usually incomplete nature of realignment may be explained by structural limits (arising from the evolutionary history of the organism) and processing limits (arising from interactions among the several adaptive processes evoked by prism exposure).

Chapter 4

PARADIGM AND GENERALIZATIONS

Prism adaptation is a surprisingly enduring subject of research. Beginning with the work of Helmholtz (1909/1962) in Germany and Stratton (1896, 1897a, 1897b) in the United States, prism adaptation was a minor but persistent research area until the systematic work of Kohler (1951/1964) at Innsbruck, Austria and Held (1961, 1968) in the United States that produced an intense flurry of research in the 1960s and 1970s (for reviews, see Rock, 1966; Welch, 1978, 1986). This momentum has abated somewhat, but still the prism adaptation paradigm is frequently used to investigate problems of perceptual and perceptual–motor plasticity.[1]

For almost 100 years, behavioral scientists have been fascinated by the ability of people to successfully deal with distortion of the visual world produced by looking through optical elements like prisms. A wide variety of optical distortions have been investigated, including lateral displacement, frontal–planar rotation, curvature, spectral refraction, magnification, and minification (see Howard, 1982; Welch, 1978). Other kinds of stimulus distortion such as that of auditory localization have also been studied (McLaughlin & Bower, 1965; Mikaelian, 1972, 1974; Radeau & Bertelson, 1977, 1978).

The term *prism adaptation* is something of a misnomer, because a variety of optical and nonoptical distortions have been studied. *Adaptation to rearrangement* is perhaps a more appropriate appellation (Welch, 1974). Nevertheless, we use the term because it is widely recognized and because it appropriately captures the scope of the present concern.

The persistent popularity is due to the methodological advantages of the paradigm, as well as to the extensive perceptual–motor plasticity that the research revealed. The prism adaptation paradigm is one of the earliest instances of black-box analysis. A prismatic transform is a known, quantifiable perturbation of system input. Observation of behavioral response to such change in stimulus input enables inferences about the intervening processes that normally map stimuli onto responses. Our ability to identify and analyze intervening processes has increased

---

[1]For recent examples of the prism adaptation paradigm see Bedford (1993a), Jakobson and Goodale (1989), Radeau (1994), Rossetti and Koga (1994), and Rossetti, Koga, and Mano (1993).

enormously in recent years, but the prism adaptation paradigm still fits comfortably in this general methodological strategy (Bedford, 1989, 1993a, 1993b).

Adaptive spatial alignment, in particular, is not well illuminated by methods normally employed to investigate strategic perceptual–motor control and motor learning. The most common source of spatial misalignment, normal drift, is relatively slow to occur (Howard, 1982; Robinson, 1976) and the contribution of realignment processes is likely to be negligible in studies of motor control that involve performance over minutes or at most hours. Even in studies of skill acquisition of longer duration, the small realignments normally necessary are likely to be obscured by more salient strategic control processes. A similar situation exists in studies of perceptual–motor development in which realignment required by growth (Bullock & Grossberg, 1988; Held & Bossom, 1961) can be confounded by perceptual–motor learning. Thus, perceptual–motor coordination under normal conditions is unlikely to tell us much about transformation processes. Misalignments arising from pathology are potentially informative (Goodale, Milner, Jakobson, & Carey, 1990; Jakobson & Goodale, 1989), but the source and nature of such dysfunctions are not yet well understood. Only investigations in situations that involve a large misalignment of known kind and onset are likely to be very informative of adaptive alignment.

In this chapter we first review the salient features of the prism adaptation paradigm, with particular emphasis on experimental control in this methodology. Then, several of the principal results obtained using this paradigm are listed as the empirical generalizations that shaped the development of the model given in chapters 5 and 6.

EXPERIMENTAL PARADIGM

General features of the prism adaptation paradigm are illustrated in Fig. 4.1. *Exposure* to the prismatic distortion is preceded and followed by observation periods during which sensory input is undistorted. The *training task* is performed with full sensory *feedback and knowledge of results* to enable adaptation to the prismatic distortion. Onset of the training task may precede the exposure period to provide a baseline from which the *direct effect* of the distortion on the training task may be assessed. Change in the direct effect over the exposure period provides a direct measure of prism adaptation. Similarly, offset of the training task may be delayed beyond the exposure period to enable direct assessment of *recovery* from prism adaptation.

Traditionally, the training task is preceded and followed by a *criterion task*, performed without distortion of sensory input and without sensory feedback or knowledge of results. Usually, only visual feedback is limited during performance of the criterion task, but attempts are sometimes made to limit proprioceptive feedback from the involved motor system(s). The criterion task may be similar to the training task or it may be selected to involve only a subset of the total perceptual–motor functions of the training task.

PRISM ADAPTATION PARADIGM

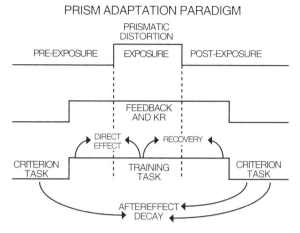

FIG. 4.1. Prism adaptation paradigm. Parallel time lines are shown for exposure to the prismatic distortion, availability of feedback and knowledge of results (KR), and administration of criterion and training tasks. Direct effects and recovery measures are illustrated as change in training task performance. Aftereffects and decay measures are illustrated as change in criterion task performance.

Change in criterion task performance from pre-exposure to postexposure provides an *aftereffect* measure of transfer of prism adaptation when (visual) feedback and knowledge of results are no longer available. Repeated postexposure application of the criterion task provides a measure of the *decay* of prism aftereffects. When criterion and training tasks are also otherwise dissimilar, aftereffects further identify involvement in prism adaptation of particular part(s) of the perceptual–motor functions exercised by the training task.

For both training and criterion tasks, the kind of change in performance that would be adaptive can be identified by the selective nature of the prismatic distortion. Typically, performance is only measured in terms of performance relative to some objective standard (e.g., target). However, kinematic performance measures are also possible.

A typical realization of the prism adaptation paradigm, for example, involves the training task of pointing at visual targets with the hand under lateral displacement of the visual field. A criterion task may be similar target pointing with the unseen limb, but other criterion tasks may be pointing straight ahead without vision or adjusting a visual stimulus to straight ahead without movement of body parts. Direct effects provide a measure of prism adaptation in terms of reduction in pointing errors that are initially made in the direction of the displacement. Recovery measures reflect a similar reduction in error, but initially in the direction opposite the preceding displacement.

Adaptive aftereffects for criterion tasks of target pointing with the unseen limb or pointing straight ahead without vision are indicated by errors opposite the direction of the previous displacement, but the adaptive error is in the same direction as the previous displacement for the criterion task of adjusting a visual stimulus to straight ahead without body movement.

Kinematic measures are also possible for both training and criterion tasks. These include changes in limb and eye movement paths and trajectories.

Direct effects include contributions to prism adaptation of adaptive changes in perceptual functions or motor functions. For example, with a training task that requires eye–hand coordination under optical displacement of the visual field, the performance error produced by misperception of visual location can be reduced by realignment of visual space and proprioceptive limb space (see chapter 2). Performance error can also be reduced by strategic motor control that, for example, deploys online control with visual feedback or utilizes knowledge of results for offline reprogramming of a feedforward movement plan to produce a more appropriate limb movement (see chapter 1). Performance during prism exposure can also be improved by motor learning of, for example, a feedforward movement plan specific to the prism exposure situation (see chapter 3). Recovery measures must also be viewed as involving all of these kinds of adaptive functions.

Aftereffects, however, provide a means of isolating the adaptive changes in perceptual function(s) that occurred during prism exposure with the training task. Because the criterion task is dissimilar to the training task, motor control strategies that are specific to the training task and associative motor learning that occurred during prism exposure are unlikely to transfer to criterion task performance. Nonassociative learning of parameter adjustments for the transformations that mediate alignment among the several intrinsic spatial representations (i.e., adaptive spatial alignment), however, is not limited to the training domain (see chapter 2). They may appear undiminished in aftereffect measures of prism adaptation. Decay of aftereffects can also be viewed as a measure of the persistence of adaptive change in perceptual functions.

The prism adaptation paradigm includes the capacity to identify the several kinds of contributors to prism adaptation. Aftereffects are especially useful in identifying the contributions of adaptive spatial alignment, and the technologies of motor control research (e.g., kinematic analysis) are increasingly applied to direct effects to identify the contributions of strategic perceptual–motor control[2] and motor learning (Jakobson & Goodale, 1989; Rossetti & Koga, 1994; Rossetti et al., 1993). The full potential of the paradigm, however, cannot be realized without explicit comparison of aftereffects and direct effects (Redding & Wallace, 1993).

GENERALIZATIONS

Six generalizations from prism adaptation research constrain the theory of adaptive spatial alignment presented in the next chapter. Any general theory that proposes to include spatial transformation processes within its domain must be capable of explaining these basic conclusions.

---

[2]Incidentally, to call strategic control *conscious correction* (e.g., Harris, 1963, 1965), is to completely misrepresent the nature and importance of these contributions to prism adaptation. Our understanding of motor control has advanced so far as to make such a term of dismissal and denigration both misleading and counterproductive.

Direct Effects Versus Aftereffects

The larger part of prism adaptation is usually accomplished by strategic perceptual–motor control, and perhaps motor learning, rather than adaptive spatial alignment. The basis for this conclusion is the widely recognized, but infrequently documented observation that performance during prism exposure (i.e., direct effects) shows rapid and usually complete error correction, whereas aftereffect measures change slowly and are usually asymptotic far short of complete compensation for the prismatic distortion (Baily, 1972; Redding & Wallace, 1993).[3] However, as illustrated in Fig. 4.2, with continued development of aftereffects, direct effects may show an overcompensation for the prismatic distortion that declines with continued exposure. The difference between direct effects and aftereffects suggests that strategic control and adaptive alignment converge to produce adaptive performance during prism exposure.

Thus, strategic control and adaptive alignment both contribute to prism adaptation. Any theory must be able to explain not only the usually limited nature of spatial realignment but also why any realignment occurs at all in the face of the higher level of compensation achieved by strategic control alone.

Spatial Discordance Versus Error Feedback

The error signal that drives spatial realignment is fundamentally different from that which drives strategic control and motor learning. This conclusion follows from the previously noted difference in relative magnitude between aftereffects and direct effects (Generalization 1) and from the further observation that error feedback is sufficient, but not necessary, for prism aftereffects (Welch, 1978). Aftereffect evidence of realignment can occur without any noticeable performance error,[4] although error feedback enhances realignment aftereffects (Coren, 1966; Welch & Abel, 1970; Welch & Rhoades, 1969). Moreover, realignment aftereffects can appear even in the face of persistent error in performance of the exposure task (Redding, Rader, & Lucas, 1992).

Therefore, *spatial discordance* that drives realignment is somehow separable from performance error. Indeed, if realignment were driven by the same kind of error signal involved in strategic control, our perception of spatial position should be constantly changing with everyday performance errors.

Figure 4.3 illustrates the logical difficulty with error feedback as a basis for spatial realignment. Successful eye–hand coordination under exposure to lateral displacement, for example, does not remove the spatial discordance between eye and hand. For an objectively straight-ahead target viewed under lateral displace-

---

[3]To our knowledge, the only instances of complete compensation in aftereffects came from Held's laboratory (Held & Bossom, 1961; Mikaelian & Held, 1964).

[4]The numerous instances of aftereffects without performance error include Dewar (1971), Howard (1967, 1982), Howard, Anstis, and Lucia (1974), Jacobson and Goodale (1989), Templeton, Howard, and Wilkinson (1974), and Uhlarik (1973).

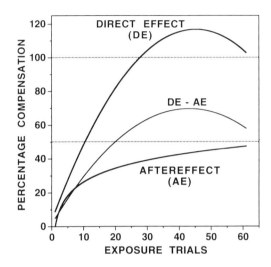

FIG. 4.2.   Direct effects and aftereffects. Idealized acquisition functions are shown for direct effect and aftereffects. The aftereffect represents realignment and the difference between direct effect and aftereffect (DE – AE) represents strategic control. Based on data from Redding and Wallace (1993, Experiment 2), in which the training task was target pointing and visual feedback first became available early in the pointing movement.

ment, target acquisition (i.e., zero error) requires that eye and hand be positioned differently in their respective coordinate systems. Strategic control processes can, and most assuredly do, contribute to improved performance during prism exposure, but such error reduction cannot remove the spatial misalignment between eye and hand. The spatial difference between corresponding positions for eye and hand (i.e., discordance) remains even when exposure performance is perfectly accurate and must be detected separately from performance error.

Thus, the perceptual–motor system seems to employ different error signals for strategic control and adaptive alignment (see also chapter 3). An adequate theory must not only provide for separate error signals, but also specify how the two kinds of processes combine to produce adaptive behavior.

Local Realignment and Additivity

Adaptive alignment consists of local changes *in* sensorimotor systems (Howard, 1971b, 1982; Templeton et al., 1974), rather than adaptive changes *between* sensorimotor systems (Hardt, Held, & Steinbach, 1971). That is, spatial discordance between, say, eye–head and hand–head systems is removed by change in the internal structures of one system that interpret spatial information from the other system, not by changing the control signals that are exchanged between systems.

This conclusion follows from the previously discussed need for separate error signals for adaptive alignment and strategic control (Generalization 2) but is especially supported by repeated findings of additivity of local aftereffects. The simple algebraic sum of local aftereffects found for parts of a perceptual–motor coordination loop is usually equal to the total aftereffect for that coordination loop exercised during prism exposure. If adaptive alignment were mediated directly by change in the control signals passed between systems, then the total aftereffect in a coordination loop should be greater than could be accounted for by local aftereffects in parts of the coordination loop. Indeed, local aftereffects should not occur at all if realignment were truly between systems. Figure 4.4 illustrates this generalization.

Although evidence of realignment at all of the local sites illustrated in Fig. 4.4 is incomplete (see Welch, 1978, pp. 55–59, for a review), there is now ample

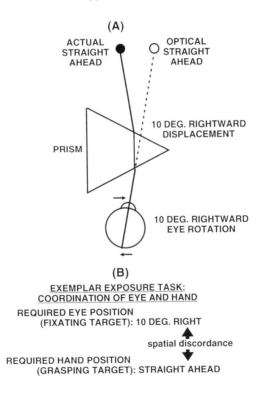

FIG. 4.3. Spatial discordance. Prismatic displacement (A) produces spatial discordance between eye and hand position (B) required to "grasp" the same physical target. Successful eye–hand coordination does not reduce this spatial discordance (redrawn from Redding & Wallace, 1992a). Reprinted from G. M. Redding and B. Wallace, "Adaptive Eye–Hand Coordination: Implications of Prism Adaptation for Perceptual–Motor Organization." In L. Proteau and D. Elliot (Eds.), *Vision and Motor Control.* Copyright 1992, p. 109, 1055 KV Amsterdam from Elsevier Science—NL, Sara Burgerhartstraat 25, 1055 KV Amsterdam, The Netherlands.

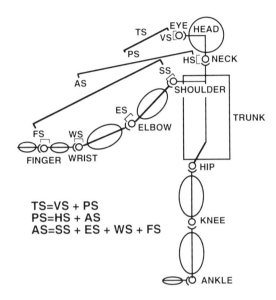

TS=VS + PS
PS=HS + AS
AS=SS + ES + WS + FS

FIG. 4.4. Hierarchy of spatial realignment. Additivity of prism aftereffects is illustrated. Total adaptive shift (TS) is equal to the sum of shifts in local spatial representations. Visual shift (VS) refers to adaptive change in the eye–head system whereas proprioceptive shift (PS) indicates change(s) in felt position from head-to-head. Head shift (HS) refers to change in felt position of the head, whereas arm shift (AS) indicates adaptive shifts in felt position of the shoulder (SS), elbow (ES), wrist (WS), or finger (FS). Similar additivity of realignment at local sites can be expected for the leg–hip system (redrawn from Redding & Wallace, 1992a). Reprinted from G. M. Redding and B. Wallace, "Adaptive Eye–Hand Coordination: Implications of Prism Adaptation for Perceptual–Motor Organization." In L. Proteau and D. Elliot (Eds.), *Vision and Motor Control.* Copyright 1992, p. 110, from Elsevier Science—NL, Sara Burgerhartstraat 25, 1055 KV Amsterdam, The Netherlands.

justification for the generalization. Aftereffect evidence of local site realignment is available for the leg–hip locomotion system (Mikaelian, 1970), the ear–head auditory system (Mikaelian, 1972, 1974), the arm–shoulder system (Hay, 1970; Hay & Brouchon, 1972), and the eye–head system (Hay & Pick, 1966b; Redding, 1978). Evidence of additivity of local aftereffects in the arm–shoulder system (i.e., AS = WS + ES + SS) has been found (Wallace & Garrett, 1975) and such additivity is especially clear in the eye–hand system.

For example, following exposure to optical displacement with an eye–hand coordination training task, three aftereffect measures are usually obtained: (a) the aftereffect measured by a criterion task of adjusting a visual target to straight ahead without body movement; (b) the aftereffect measured by a criterion task of pointing straight ahead with the unseen limb; and (c) the aftereffect measured by a criterion task of target pointing with the unseen limb. The first aftereffect reflects realignment in the eye–head system or visual shift (VS). The second aftereffect reflects realignment in the hand–head system or proprioceptive shift (PS). The third aftereffect reflects the total realignment in the eye–hand coordination loop or total shift (TS).[5] The generalization TS = VS + PS has now been verified many times.[6]

Exceptions to additivity can occur (Welch et al., 1974), but they can usually be explained by transfer to the criterion task of control strategies deployed for the training task (Redding & Wallace, 1976, 1978; Wallace & Redding, 1979) and additivity provides a converging check on the assumption that aftereffects are exclusively measures of realignment (Redding & Wallace, 1993). Moreover, the fact that aftereffects can be detected with criterion tasks that do not involve common action of the systems exercised during exposure (i.e., the training task) clearly argues against the common assumption that perceptual–motor coordination and spatial transformation are the same process.

Additivity of local aftereffects also implies a hierarchy of spatial representation (see chapter 2), whereby the reference frame of a superordinate system is built up from reference frames of subordinate systems. For example, the eye–hand reference frame is built up from eye–head and hand–head references frames. Realignment of a composite system is the sum of realignments of its components. The hierarchical relationship among local spatial representations is especially clear for the arm–shoulder system, where aftereffects at proximal joints transfer to distal joints, but not vice versa (Hay, 1970; see also Paillard, 1993b). Realignment of a superordinate component extends to subordinate components, but realignment of subordinate components contribute additively to the total realignment of the composite system.

Thus, spatial representation is hierarchically organized around sensorimotor subsystems, each of which has the capacity to adaptively transform spatial input into its own unique coordinates. Any theory of prism adaptation must be capable of explaining local alignment–realignment independent of the control signals that enable coordination of sensorimotor systems to perform more global perceptual–motor (training) tasks during prism exposure.

Variable Locus and Directional Guidance

When spatially misaligned sensorimotor systems are coordinated to perform an exposure training task, realignment is localized in the situationally subordinate system rather than the superordinate system. Although realignment is a separable part of adaptive performance during prism exposure (Generalizations 1, 2, and 3), the control strategies deployed during exposure determine the kind and amount of realignment that occurs. This conclusion is based upon interpretation of several

---

[5]The total shift aftereffect traditionally has been called the *negative aftereffect* (NA). Such usage reflects the early days of prism adaptation research when only this single aftereffect measure was obtained. The multiple aftereffect measures that are now recognized makes this terminology ambiguous.

[6]Instances of such additivity include Hay and Pick (1966b), Redding (1978), Redding and Wallace (1976, 1978), Templeton et al. (1974), Wallace (1977), Welch (1974), Welch, Choe, and Heinrich (1974), and Wilkinson (1971).

studies that varied the kind of prism aftereffect by manipulating the structure of the exposure training task (Canon, 1970; Kelso et al., 1975; Uhlarik & Canon, 1971; see also Hamilton, 1964; Howard & Templeton, 1966).

Canon (1970) required subjects to track the location of a visible sounding target with their unseen right hand. Different training tasks required subjects to track the movement of either the optically displaced visual target or the pseudophonically displaced auditory target, where the optical and auditory displacements were in opposite directions. In this manner, either the eye–head or the ear–head was the superordinate system in the sense of specifying the target for the coordination response. The other systems (eye–head or ear–head and hand–head) were subordinate in the sense of receiving rather than sending efference. Because subjects were not permitted visual feedback for the tracking response, they could not detect the misalignment between hand–head and visual or auditory systems and there was no basis for realignment of the (subordinate) hand–head response system. Subjects could, however, detect the discordance between locations in visual space and auditory space. Criterion tasks specific to change in eye–head or ear–head reference frames revealed that aftereffects were largely localized in the situationally subordinate system (eye–head or ear–head). The direction of guidance (superordinate to subordinate) specified by the different targets for pointing during prism exposure determined the locus of realignment.

In a similar study, Kelso et al. (1975) employed training tasks that required subjects to point with their unseen right hand either at an optically displaced visual target or at their own unseen left hand, whose position they were told was coincidental with the visual target. Subjects were then given verbal feedback (knowledge of results) concerning the pointing response. Thus, either the eye–head or left-hand–head was the superordinate system and the other systems (eye–head or left-hand–head and right-hand–head) were subordinate. Apparently, the subject's belief that the visual target and the proprioceptive (left hand) target occupied the same position was sufficient to evoke discordance because results were even more dramatic than those of Canon (1970). Aftereffects were entirely localized in the situationally subordinate system (eye–head or left-hand–head).[7] When the direction of guidance was eyes-to-right-hand (i.e., pointing at the visual target), the spatial discordance between positions of the visual target and the left hand produced a change in the position sense of the left hand. When the guidance was left-hand-to-right-hand, the same discordance produced a change in the position sense of the eyes.

Spatial discordance alone does not specify the source of the misalignment. Strategic control in the form of the direction of guidance linkage between misaligned sensorimotor systems is also necessary (see also discussion of the correspondence problem in chapter 3).

---

[7]Note that the offline knowledge of results provided in the Kelso et al. (1975) study probably was not directly responsible for the realignment. Discordance detection is more likely based in comparison of targeted position and the implicit position that would be necessary to achieve the target (see Redding & Wallace, 1995a, 1996a).

Uhlarik and Canon (1971) varied the direction of guidance between eye–head and hand–head systems by manipulating the availability of visual feedback. Subjects pointed at optically displaced targets with their right hand, but in different conditions, the limb was continuously visible throughout the sagittal pointing movement or only the tip of the finger was visible at the termination of the movement. In continuous exposure, subjects may depend on sight to guide the hand to the target, but in terminal exposure, subjects must depend largely on the felt position of the limb to perform the coordination task. The direction of control signals between these discordant systems is eye-to-hand for continuous exposure and hand-to-eye for terminal exposure.

Prism aftereffects were largely restricted to the situationally subordinate system: proprioceptive shift with continuous exposure and visual shift with terminal exposure (see also Redding & Wallace, 1988b). It seems that whether realignment is localized in visual or proprioceptive systems depends on the direction of the guidance linkage deployed by strategic control (see also chapter 1). Moreover, the fact that realignment is localized in the subsystem whose feedback is not utilized in control of common eye–hand action is also inconsistent with a view of performance feedback as a sufficient basis for adaptive spatial alignment.

Thus, where realignment occurs depends on the direction of control between spatially misaligned sensorimotor systems. Any theory must account for this dependence while also explaining the separable natures of adaptive spatial alignment and strategic perceptual–motor control.

Attention and Higher Level Processes

Realignment involves conscious (intentional) processes only indirectly in how perceptual–motor resources are marshaled to perform the exposure coordination task, not directly in detection and reduction of the resultant discordance. This conclusion is consistent with the repeated observation that prism aftereffects can occur without any conscious awareness of the distortion.[8] Indeed, foreknowledge of the distortion does not prevent performance error during exposure. Stronger support for this generalization comes from the observation that prism aftereffects suffer interference from a secondary cognitive task such as mental arithmetic when the exposure task involves largely controlled processing, but not when the training task involves largely automatic processing (see chapter 1).

Prism aftereffects are depressed when subjects are required to perform mental arithmetic while walking about hallways during prism exposure (Redding, Clark, & Wallace, 1985; Redding & Wallace, 1985a).[9] The optic flow necessary for walking is not distorted by prisms and automated walking is not affected by either

---

[8]Evidence of aftereffects without conscious awareness is extensive in the traditional prism adaptation literature (Howard, 1967; Howard et al., 1974; Templeton et al., 1974; Uhlarik, 1973) and has also been recently confirmed (Jakobson & Goodale, 1989).

[9]See also Barr, Schultheis, and Robinson (1976).

the prismatic distortion or the secondary cognitive task (Redding & Wallace, 1985b). Other kinds of perceptual–motor tasks, however, are affected by the distortion. For example, visual orienting of eyes and head toward a sound source or a wall encountered by the shoulder fails to exactly locate the sound or obstacle because of optical displacement. Such orienting behaviors are optional compared to the primary task of locomotion, and a secondary cognitive task interferes with such controlled processing. To the extent that the frequency of such controlled processes is reduced by cognitive load, discordance detection fails and realignment aftereffects are depressed.

In contrast, prism aftereffects are unaffected by cognitive load imposed while pointing at visual targets during prism exposure (Redding et al., 1992). The automatic components of target pointing are sufficient to place the hand in the vicinity of the target, enabling discordance detection and realignment. The more controlled processes (e.g., feedback control) involved in terminal error correction are affected by the secondary cognitive task and small errors persist during prism exposure, but automatic linkage of eye and hand is sufficient for realignment.

Thus, adaptive alignment appears to be insulated from higher level cognitive processes, but may be indirectly affected by the involvement of such processes in strategic control. Theories must account for the automatic nature of realignment while providing for the influence of controlled processes higher in the hierarchy of perceptual–motor control.

Separable Mechanisms and Modularity

Adaptive spatial alignment is realized by a variety of separable but functionally similar mechanisms rather than by a single superordinate mechanism. The modular organization (cf. Fodor, 1983; Radeau, 1994) of the perceptual–motor system is implicit in the observation that different kinds of adaptive shift occur (Generalization 3), depending on how the separate modules are coordinated (Generalization 4). Local transformational mechanisms are activated by the cooperative interaction of sensorimotor systems. Further evidence comes from the impenetrability of adaptive alignment by higher level conscious processes (Generalization 5). Higher level cognitive processes are involved only in establishing coordinative linkages among modules. But, the strongest evidence of modularity comes from the observation that adaptive alignment involves similar but separable mechanisms for different kinds of prismatic distortions. For instance, tilt and displacement aftereffects are parametrically similar even though the two kinds of adaptation do not interfere with each other (Redding, 1973a, 1973b, 1975a, 1975b).

The observation of parametrically similar, but independent aftereffects suggests that the mind–brain has solved the problem of maintaining cross-alignment among its various parts in a similar fashion. Each module includes the capacity to respond to remote realignment signals received from other modules. An adequate theory must reflect this modular organization.

IMPLICATIONS

The model developed in chapters 5 and 6 is based on the general view of perceptual–motor organization and adaptability suggested by these generalizations. The perceptual–motor system appears to be organized into distinct modules that are specialized in function. Cooperative interaction (coordination) requires a configuration of hierarchical–heterarchical linkages among the task-relevant subset of modules (i.e., strategic control). Such linkages may be automatic for habitual tasks, but nonhabitual tasks require limited central processing capacity to establish and maintain the required linkage.

Adaptive alignment is the process that normally maintains spatial cross-alignment among the various modules in the face of naturally occurring misalignments arising from growth, pathology, or drift. Separate, but similar mechanisms residing in each module serve to locally realign the module in response to a remote, guiding signal from another module. The multiple directions of linkage required by the variety of everyday coordination assures that the various components of the perceptual–motor system are maintained in a veridical state of cross-alignment (see also Craske, 1975).

The prism adaptation paradigm is uniquely suited to studying adaptive spatial alignment, but such experimentally introduced misalignment also evokes the full adaptive capacity of the perceptual–motor system. Any theory of adaptive spatial alignment must also acknowledge the contributions of strategic control and motor learning to adaptive performance.

Chapter 5

CONTRIBUTIONS OF STRATEGIC CONTROL

The prism adaptation paradigm evokes in the perceptual–motor system both ordinary and extraordinary adaptive capacities. Ordinary capacity for rapid adaptive performance in the face of normal imprecision in perceptual and motor processes: extraordinary capacity for gradual adaptive adjustment in the spatial mapping functions that enable spatial alignment among internal representations. Because misalignment among spatial representations produces performance error, exposure to prismatic distortion evokes ordinary adaptive processes. In this chapter, we sketch a model of perceptual–motor performance in which the contributions of ordinary adaptive processes to prism adaptation can be understood.

First, we define the organizational units of the perceptual–motor system, suggesting autonomy, orienting function, and structural contiguity as defining characteristics of these basic sensorimotor systems. Then, we discuss the issues of guidance linkages, control signals, and planning in the coordination of basic systems to produce functionally larger systems. Finally, we show how feedback control and feedforward control, based on knowledge of results and associative learning, can compensate for performance errors produced by prismatic distortions. We conclude that, although ordinary strategic control and associative learning can produce adaptive performance during prism exposure, such adaptation does not address the more fundamental problem of spatial alignment and realignment.

BASIC SENSORIMOTOR SYSTEMS

The review of perceptual–motor performance in chapter 1 suggests that semi-autonomous sensorimotor systems are the basic organizational units of the perceptual–motor system (see Fig. 1.2). The present model attributes prism adaptation partly to control processes that strategically coordinate sensorimotor systems adaptively to perform the exposure training task (see chapter 4; Generalization 1) and partly to spatial mapping processes that restore spatial alignment among sensorimotor systems (see chapter 4; Generalization 2). We begin, therefore, by considering the nature of these basic sensorimotor systems: first some defining characteristics and then some illustrative examples.

The concept of a sensorimotor system satisfies what we believe is a fundamental requirement for any theory of human performance—namely, the interdependence of perceptual and motor functions. It is a truism that perception without action is meaningless. Indeed, it can be argued that motor performance is the *raison d'être* for perception, that the brain is chiefly a device for sensorimotor control and only incidentally a device for knowledge acquisition (Churchland, 1986; Rozin, 1976). Moreover, the human brain evolved from earlier kinds of brains that served simpler perceptual–motor functions (e.g., feeding, striking, fleeing). Therefore, the brain may be viewed as an evolutionary collection of modules (cf. Fodor, 1983) that serve specialized perceptual–motor functions and that are structurally constrained to minimize wiring and maximize speed of communication among neurons working in concert (Kupferman, 1981). Cooperative interaction of these modules to enable more molar perceptual–motor functions may be the evolutionarily more recent aspect of perceptual–motor organization. This view of perceptual–motor organization suggests certain logical requirements for the primitive organizational units.

Defining Characteristics

First, a module should be capable of autonomous spatial behavior, having the sensory and motor capacities sufficient for stimulus encoding and response execution independent of any other module (see also chapter 1). Hence, we call these modules *sensorimotor systems,* the subsystems of the total perceptual–motor system. The term *sensorimotor* is intended to convey the idea of subsets of the larger perceptual–motor category. *Sensory capacity* includes the ability to encode distal attributes of extrapersonal space (i.e., exteroceptors). *Motor capacity* is the ability to execute a response appropriate to the information coded by an exteroceptor. A sensorimotor system should also include sensors (i.e., proprioceptors) for the current position of its effector in interpersonal space. Thus, sensorimotor systems consist of exteroceptors, effectors, and proprioceptors, with control structures to support specialized functions (see Fig. 1.2).

A corollary of autonomy is the capacity of sensorimotor systems to operate independently, without mutual interference, and, in the extreme, to produce *contradictory behavior.* That such conflict (e.g., misalignment) may ultimately be resolved (e.g., realignment) only reinforces the point that the systems are separable at some lower level of organization. The fact that such conflict resolution consists of altering the local function of one or the other system rather than some higher order function relating the systems (chapter 4; Generalization 3) clearly indicates the primacy of the basic sensorimotor systems.

Second, the simplest kinds of sensorimotor systems are orienting systems. Exploration of and information pickup from extrapersonal space may be the most primitive kind of specialized function. Such systems work to direct more or less narrowly focused exteroceptors to different points in extrapersonal space. Here, the exteroceptor is attached to its effector, so it moves with effector movement. In this case, proprioceptors may serve the additional function of extending the range of exteroceptive function by providing for integration of successive exteroceptor inputs to create an extended spatial representation. Because the exteroceptor is attached to the effector, proprioceptor output provides the basis for mapping exteroceptor inputs onto a locus in body-centric space. Such orienting functions would appear to be a prerequisite to any manipulation of the environment. Indeed, manipulation systems may be another level of organization, involving coordination of more primitive, orienting sensorimotor systems.

Third, the various components of a sensorimotor system should be structurally contiguous. An organizational unit should minimize the length of neural connections among its sensory and motor elements that work cooperatively. Speed of communication among neurons that work together is, therefore, maximized. Moreover, for orienting systems in which the effector serves to move the exteroceptor in extrapersonal space, the elements of a sensorimotor system should be physiologically contiguous. Thus, consideration of physiological function can provide an approximation of a sensorimotor system in lieu of detailed neuroanatomical data about connectivity.

The complexity of the perceptual–motor system makes the task of identifying components something of a bootstrap operation. In order to devise tests of the independence of sensorimotor systems one must first be able to identify the systems. The heuristics of autonomous operation, orienting function, and structural contiguity provide an edge to break into this problem of circularity. Application of these heuristics is illustrated in the following examples.

Illustrations

Figure 5.1 identifies some sensorimotor systems suggested by the review of prism adaptation research in chapter 4, especially the evidence of autonomous operation (i.e., contradictory behavior) given by local realignment and additivity (Generalization 3), which we believe to be among the best available behavioral indicators of modular systems. Only if two systems are separable can they be made to show contradictory behavior. In the present section, we focus on describing how each system may function independently and defer consideration of the coordinative linkages among systems until the next section.

The structural unit *eye-to-head* may be a specialized system for orienting to points in head-centric space. When we sit quietly reading, the eye–head functions are largely independent of any other system. The narrow (foveal) focus of the retina (exteroceptor) is moved about by the extraocular muscles (effector) and the eye position sense (proprioceptor[1]) provides a basis for integrating foveal input in extended visual space.

The structural unit *ear-to-neck* may be a specialized system for orienting to points in trunk-centric space. When we turn our head to localize an unseen sound

---

[1]We defer consideration of the nature of the eye position sense until discussion of spatial mapping in chapter 6, in which the distinction between inflow and outflow becomes critical.

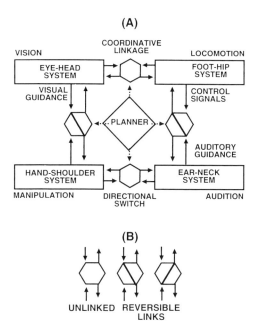

FIG. 5.1. Basic sensorimotor systems (A) and coordinative linkages (B). Basic systems may function autonomously (unlinked) or they may be coordinated (linked) via directional switches set by higher level planning functions that respond to overall task organization. The linkages shown are such that locomotion (foot–hip) and manipulation (hand–shoulder) systems are guided by visual (eye–head) and auditory (ear–neck) systems, respectively, but linkages may be reversed for less common coordination tasks.

source, the ear–neck system can function independently. This system especially illustrates the facilitative cooperation of sensory and motor functions. Imprecision in difference signals between the two ears may be reduced by moving the head (and ears) to minimize differences and utilization of the head position sense to better localize the source in auditory space. The eye position sense may similarly compensate for imprecise peripheral localization in the visual system.

The *hand-to-shoulder* structural unit may be a specialized system for exploring trunk-centric space. When we scratch ourselves, adjust clothing without looking, or explore our bedside table in the dark, the hand–shoulder is largely free of external influence from other sensorimotor systems. The narrow focus of tactile sensors in the fingers (exteroceptor) is moved about by the limb muscles (effector), and the limb position sense (proprioceptor) provides the basis for positioning the hand in the extended limb space.

When we negotiate our bedroom in the dark, the *foot-to-hip* system may function in a manner that is largely independent of other systems. Tactile sensors may provide information about characteristics of the walking surface and obstacles encountered by the moving limb that may then be integrated to form an extended representation of limb space.

Note that a given physiological structure may serve more than one sensorimotor function. For example, the eye–head structure may include separate systems for processing location, orientation, and motion information. Different exteroceptor functions for encoding location of retinal stimulation, retinal orientation of an extended stimulus, and direction of movement of an image across the retina may be uniquely connected with effector–proprioceptor functions of the extraocular muscles, thereby producing parallel and largely independent systems for orienting to stimulus location, scanning stimulus orientation, and tracking stimulus movement in head-centric space.

We offer these examples as tentative illustrations of basic or natural kinds of sensorimotor systems, the primitive perception–action units endowed by evolution. Although these units are suggested by prism adaptation research and other kinds of data (see chapter 1), our knowledge of basic sensorimotor systems is far from complete. Perhaps the greatest challenge is to distinguish such basic systems from functional systems that arise from the hierarchical organization of basic systems to deal with consistently occurring environmental tasks. In the following section, we discuss such coordination of basic systems to form functional systems.

COORDINATION
(FUNCTIONAL SENSORIMOTOR SYSTEMS)

By *coordination* we mean common action of basic sensorimotor systems. Autonomous operation of sensorimotor systems can produce many types of specialized (e.g., orienting) perceptual–motor behavior. But many, if not most, perceptual–motor tasks require that systems be functionally linked in a coordinated fashion (e.g., manipulation). Such coordination tasks are sufficiently general in scope to generate functional sensorimotor systems with certain general characteristics. Here we discuss three such characteristics: the hierarchical nature of (guidance) linkages between basic sensorimotor systems, the kinds of (control) signals that may be exchanged between basic systems, and the role of higher level (planning) processes in coordination.

Guidance

Figure 5.1 illustrates some of the more intuitive coordinative linkages. Note that the direction of linkage between systems can be reversed from that shown and systems can also be unlinked for autonomous operation. For example, reaching for an object may be largely accomplished by visual (eye–head system) control of the proprioceptive (hand–shoulder) system, but proprioceptively controlled looking also occurs, as when we direct our eyes to read our wrist watch or to look at an object we have just touched. Similarly, locomotion (foot–hip system) is usually under visual control, but an irregularity in pavement can reverse the direction of linkage, causing us to look toward our feet.

We characterize these cooperative connections among sensorimotor systems as *unidirectional guidance linkages*, which permit the transfer of spatially coded instructions among systems. For example, in visually guided reaching, the visual target position transferred to the limb is a command to move the limb to that position. In visually guided locomotion, visual movement information constitutes a signal to adjust the direction of locomotion. The direction of coordinative linkage may be strategically reversed, but a given system cannot simultaneously be guiding and be guided by another system. Thus, coordinative linkage of sensorimotor systems is hierarchical in nature: For any given linkage, there is at least one superordinate (guiding) system and at least one subordinate (guided) system. But, superordinate–subordinate relationships can be heterarchically reversed.

A guided system may nevertheless enjoy a certain amount of autonomy. For example, a guiding system may simply specify a movement goal that selects a feedforward movement plan in the guided system. Execution of the selected movement plan may then be a purely local concern of the guided system, employing locally available sensory information for predictive (feedforward) control and error-corrective (feedback) control. Alternatively, if the guiding system has exteroceptor access to the behavior of the guided (controlled) system, predictive and error-corrective control may be more continuously exercised by the guiding system.

Interaction among sensorimotor systems is for purposes of cooperative action. Thus, information exchange is in the form of *control signals*. There is no direct exchange of purely sensory information. A guiding system's exteroceptor is its only possible source of purely sensory information about the guided system. Spatial information directly exchanged between systems is couched in terms of control signals designed to produce common action of sensorimotor systems. Knowledge structures (i.e., spatial representation) develop from such cooperative action and are to be explained in terms of their control function.

Control Signals

The directional nature of guidance linkages and the prohibition on direct exchange of sensory information between coordinatively linked sensorimotor systems places limits on the control signals that can be used in the coordination of sensorimotor systems. Two kinds of control signals can be distinguished (see Fig. 5.2), depending on the manner in which spatial information is represented (see also chapter 2) and on their control function (see also chapter 1).

Position codes represent spatial information in terms of coordinates centered on the most proximal articulation of a sensorimotor system. For example, a targeted visual position (eye–head system) is represented in the head-centric coordinates of visual space and a targeted proprioceptive limb position (hand–shoulder system) is represented in body-centric coordinates of limb space.

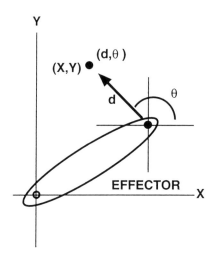

FIG. 5.2.   Movement control codes. Effector movement may be controlled by *position codes* (x,y), which represent target information in terms of coordinates centered on the most proximal articulation of the effector, or by *difference codes* (d, θ), which represent target information in terms of coordinates centered on the present position of the effector endpoint.

Difference codes represent spatial information in terms of a coordinate system centered on present position of an effector. For example, a targeted visual position is represented relative to present eye position in visual space (eye–head system) and a targeted proprioceptive position is represented relative to present limb position in limb space (hand–shoulder system).

Position codes are particularly well-suited to offline specification of initial conditions in feedforward control of movement. The position of a target can be used to select an optimal feedforward movement plan without also having to specify initial position of the controlled effector. At the kinematic level, the movement plan consists in a predictable sequence of positions for the controlled effector derived by extrapolating backward from targeted position to initial position (Bullock & Grossberg, 1988; Bullock et al., 1993). At the dynamic level, the movement plan consists in a predictable sequence of patterned agonist–antagonist activation derived by backward extrapolation from relative activation required to achieve the targeted position to relative activation for the initial position. At all levels, available afference can be monitored to detect early evidence of impending, predictable disturbances.

Position codes might also be used for online feedback control, but this amounts to recoding the error as a difference between present effector position and targeted position (i.e., difference coding), at least when coordinated systems are spatially misaligned. For example, a visible error in limb positioning that occurs with visual guidance and optical displacement of the visual field cannot be corrected by reissuing a command expressing the target position. Such a command would simply continue the error. Performance can be improved by redefining the position of the target, but this amounts to offline correction based in knowledge of results, not online feedback correction (see also chapter 1).

Difference coding is the natural kind of movement coding in feedback control. The position of a target relative to present effector position is a direct expression of the spatial difference (error) that must be reduced in order for the effector to achieve the target. Kinematically, the required movement is represented as a spatial vector specifying direction and magnitude. Dynamically, the required movement is represented as a timed impulse specifying muscle activation level and duration. At all levels, available feedback can be used to correct for unpredictable disturbances (i.e., errors).

Difference codes have also be used for representation in feedforward movement plans (Crossman & Goodeve, 1963/1983; Kawato, Isobe, Maeda, & Suzuki, 1988; Keele, 1968; Meyer et al., 1988; Schmidt et al., 1979), but our assumption that purely sensory signals are not passed between sensorimotor systems makes this an unlikely possibility, at least for coordination of sensorimotor systems. For example, in the case of visual guidance for which the controlled limb is not visible, starting position of the limb is not available and difference movement codes cannot be calculated (but see Rossetti, Desmurget, & Prablanc, 1995). Limb position in proprioceptive space might be made available as a control signal to the eyes, but this requires reversing the direction of guidance between limb and eyes. If the limb is visible, starting limb position in visual space is available, but in this case it seems more likely that visual guidance of the limb would depend on feedback control to reduce the spatial difference between limb and target (i.e., difference coding). Moreover, because many sensorimotor systems lack exteroceptive access to other systems (e.g., the tactile sense provides no information about visual position), it seems unlikely that movement plans are generally couched in terms of difference codes.

Substantial evidence favors difference (vector) codes over position codes. A variety of psychophysical studies (Bonnet, Requin, & Stelmach, 1982; Favilla, Hening, & Ghez, 1989; Rosenbaum, 1980; Soechting & Terzuolo, 1990), neurophysiological studies (Fu, Suarez, & Ebner, 1993; Georgopoulos, Kalaska, Caminiti, & Massey, 1982; Schwartz, Kettner, & Georgopolous, 1988), and simulation studies (Bullock & Grossberg, 1988; Bullock et al., 1993) suggest that the control of movement involves distinct coding (parameterization or parcellation) of distance and direction, that distance and direction are not locked together in a location code. Moreover, horizontal movement may be controlled by codes that are distinct from codes for either vertical movements or distance movements (Flanders & Soechting, 1990; Grobstein, 1988).

However, evidence of parcellation does not exclude position codes from a role in motor control (see also Fu et al., 1993; Grobstein, 1988). Parameterization of movement for the different spatial dimensions may reflect the activity of hypothetical pattern generators that are specialized for different planes of movement and that are selected from "a more general signal representing stimulus location in three-dimensional space" (Grobstein, 1988, p. 40). Distinct coding of directions and distance could apply at the level of motor circuitry (pattern generators), but position coding could describe a higher level of spatial representation involved in movement planning (see also Morasso, 1981; Soechting, 1989). Such circuitry could be suited for executing movements both with efficient corrective adjustments along selected dimensions under feedback control and with complete position specification under feedforward control (see also, Bullock & Grossberg, 1988; Bullock et al., 1993).

For these reasons, we make the strong assumption that, at least between basic sensorimotor systems, feedforward control is expressed in terms of signals that represent spatial position and feedback control signals express differences in spatial position. Feedforward and feedback control are served by different channels. Moreover, we demonstrate in chapter 6 that such a distinction between movement codes is necessary for detection of spatial misalignment and realignment of sensorimotor systems.

Planning

Coordinative linkage of basic systems to select (or create) a functional sensorimotor system requires higher level decision processes that are strategically sensitive to particular task demands. We represent selection of a task-dependent organization by the centrally located *planner* in Fig. 5.1. We consider this planner to be the principal source of strategic (task-sensitive) flexibility in perceptual–motor performance, but it is also the principal locus of limited processing capacity (Generalization 5, chapter 4). Strategic control is, therefore, limited by processing load. In the following discussion of planner operation, we first distinguish at least three ways in which the variety and complexity of everyday coordination tasks may impose large processing loads. Then, we consider how this load may be reduced. Figure 5.1 is, of course, an extreme simplification. Many of the linkages and basic systems we discuss subsequently are not shown explicitly in this figure.

First, coordination tasks often require task-dependent *guidance reversals* between basic sensorimotor systems. For example, when vision is partially obscured by obstacles, we work alternately by feel and by sight (e.g., sewing and automobile repair). The following laboratory analog of such tasks illustrates how strategic reversal in coordinative linkage may also involve change in the kind of control signal that is passed between basic systems.

When sight of the hand is possible only for the terminal part of a reaching movement (i.e., terminally closed-loop), movement may be initiated in a feedforward manner by a control signal to the limb (visual guidance) that expresses the position of the visual target. Before the moving limb becomes visible and before visual feedback control of the limb is possible, the hand–shoulder system may operate autonomously to execute the movement plan selected by the initial control signal from the eye–head system. That is, the two systems may be unlinked, but more likely, the direction of guidance may be reversed, with the eye tracking the moving limb. Because purely sensory (proprioceptive) information about limb position is assumed not to be directly available, such proprioceptive guidance of the eyes would consist of a series of positions of the moving limb sent as control signals for feedforward execution of saccadic eye movements to fixate successive limb positions.[2] Now, when the limb becomes visible, two kinds of changes in movement control should occur. The discrepancy (difference code) between fovea and hand should elicit an error-corrective saccadic movement to fixate the hand. Also, the visible discrepancy (difference code) between hand and target should reinstitute visual guidance of the limb (feedback control) to correct the error so that the hand can achieve the target.

Planning for this hypothetical performance would involve two reversals in direction of linkage (between visual eye–head and proprioceptive hand–shoulder systems) and two types of movement control channels (position and difference codes), and linkage activation must be timed to coincide with particular points in the movement path. Even when the limb is continuously visible, the initial movement may be controlled in a feedforward manner, but the terminal part of the movement path may be under feedback control, and movement planning must be sensitive to speed and accuracy demands of the particular task (see chapter 1).

Second, coordination tasks often require *alternating guidance* of one sensorimotor system by two (or more) other systems. For example, silencing the alarm clock with the hand(s) may be accomplished by alternate signals from the sleep-hooded eyes and the irritated ears; walking in a darkened room may be alternately guided by vision and the sound shadows cast by furniture and walls. These examples also illustrate the need for habitual visual guidance to be overridden when faced with degraded visual information. Alternate guidance requires that the planner evaluate the competing control signals.

Third, coordination tasks often require *simultaneous guidance* of two (or more) systems by another system. For example, when we use both hands on the morning cup of coffee, simultaneous visual guidance of both hands is required; walking in a darkened room and searching movements of the hand(s) may be simultaneously guided by sound shadows (or alternately by vision). Obviously, simultaneously guided systems must also be timed to work together. Simultaneous guidance requires that the planner synchronize control signals.

Simultaneous guidance is more ubiquitous than might be supposed from the coarse level of representation illustrated in Fig. 5.1. Even apparently simple tasks may involve multiple target attributes (e.g., location, orientation, size, and shape) with distributed control along parallel channels, each channel controlling a different aspect of the response of the guided system (Arbib, 1981). Thus, each linkage between sensorimotor systems shown in Fig. 5.1 should be considered to be composed of a number of parallel and perhaps largely independent channels, each concerned with a different component of perceptual–motor behavior. For instance, when we reach for a visual object, the transportation (reaching) component is parameterized for target characteristics such as size and distance, whereas the manipulation (grip formation and grasping) component is guided by the visual shape and orientation of the target, and the two components are synchronized to

---

[2]Unlike tracking the visible limb, for which the position of the eye (fovea) relative to the limb is available for continuous control of pursuit movements, tracking the nonvisible limb should involve discrete control of saccadic movements.

facilitate achievement of their respective goals (Jeannerod, 1981, 1984, 1986a, 1986b; Jeannerod & Biguer, 1982).

Movement channels in peripheral vision have also been suggested that guide the initial part of the trajectory in visually guided reaching (Paillard, 1980, 1982; Paillard, Jordon, & Brouchon, 1981). Similar movement channels, sensitive to Gibson like optical flow patterns (Gibson, 1966, 1979; Hildreth, 1984a, 1984b; Longuet-Higgins & Prazdny, 1980), have been suggested to guide walking (Fitch, Tuller, & Turvey, 1982; Lee & Thomson, 1982).

Thus, in addition to multiple linkages and linkage states, perceptual–motor coordination may involve multiple, parallel channels and a timed sequence of linkage states for multiple intersystem linkages. Such strategic flexibility places heavy demands on central processing (programming) capacity (Klein, 1976; Stelmach, 1982). We assume a limited capacity for intentional control of coordinative linkages (Posner & Snyder, 1975; Schneider & Shiffrin, 1977a) that must be circumvented to avoid coordination failure. The skilled actor has acquired (learned) the ability to minimize processing load on the planner in two ways: the formation of coordinative structures (synergies), which effectively reduces the number of linkages that must be controlled and automation, which largely removes a linkage from planner control.

A *coordinative structure* (Bernstein, 1967; see also Tuller, Turvey, & Fitch, 1982) means that two (or more) sensorimotor systems (e.g., reaching and grasping movements of the hand or the complex of movements and postural adjustments involved in walking) are constrained to operate simultaneously as a single unit and, in effect, a single linkage setting can transfer multiple target attributes (e.g., location and orientation) from guiding to guided systems. Note that the two movement components are synchronized (Jeannerod, 1981, 1984, 1986a, 1986b; Jeannerod & Biguer, 1982), and any accommodation to feedback requires that the combined movement be timed by the slower of the two components (Kelso et al., 1979).

Automation (e.g., Hasher & Zacks, 1979) means that the task- relevant sequence of switch settings is situationally preselected and the required behavior runs off in the absence of an inhibiting signal from the planner. Habitual and highly skilled behavior (e.g., walking and catching) are largely under feedforward control, with each step in the program triggering the next, and do not require continuous feedback monitoring by the guiding system (Arbib, 1972; Kelso, 1982). Behaviors that are sufficiently important (and repetitious) to become automated are usually also sufficiently complex to require a coordinative structure, but coordinative structures can also be utilized in nonautomated control (Kelso et al., 1979).

Planning is influenced by the overall task organization, including explicit or implicit instructions, the available processing capacity (e.g., whether multiple tasks must be performed simultaneously), and the availability of a sensorimotor system to serve as a guiding source (e.g., vision may not be available because it is entirely or partially occluded). However, planner operation is also influenced by a variety of memorial factors, including available coordinative structures together with knowledge of their structural limits (e.g., precision, accuracy, and reaction time) as applied to the specific task and available automated procedures along with their habit strength in a given task situation.

Clearly, understanding perceptual–motor performance requires that we go beyond the nominal task organization to a consideration of the structures and processes linking sensorimotor systems. In the next section we consider how the perceptual–motor system so conceived can respond adaptively to the challenge posed by artificially induced spatial misalignment among its component parts.

STRATEGIC CONTROL AND ASSOCIATIVE LEARNING

We identify three ways in which ordinary adaptive perceptual–motor processes can be deployed to compensate for performance error induced by spatial misalignment of hierarchically linked sensorimotor systems: feedback control based in online error feedback, feedforward control based in offline knowledge of results, and associative learning of feedforward control based in contingent input–output relationships. Figure 5.3 illustrates the following discussion of strategic control and associative learning; however, the reader may also refer to the more expanded

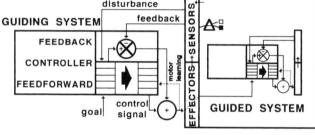

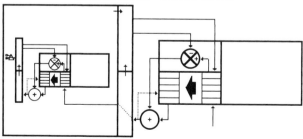

FIG. 5.3. Adaptive coordination. Directional guidance linkages establish a guiding (controlling) system and a guided (controlled) system. Control signals are sent both to the effectors of the guiding system and to the controller(s) of the guided system. Compensation for performance error induced by spatial misalignment between systems can be achieved in the guiding system by feedback control (error feedback), by resetting the goal of the feedforward movement plan, or by learning a movement plan contingent on the misalignment.

illustration of motor control processes in Fig. 3.3. Because of the need to represent linkage between sensorimotor systems, Fig. 5.3 is a condensed version of Fig. 3.3.

For example, the top part of Fig. 5.3 can be taken to represent the common case of visual guidance of the hand–head, proprioceptive system by the eye–head, visual system, in which the misalignment has its source in prismatic distortion of extero-ceptor input to the guiding sensorimotor system. Performance errors arise because the existing function mapping the task–work space representation of the guiding system onto the task–work space representation of the guided system does not pick out corresponding points. For example, a goal encoded by the guiding system does not match the spatial location of guided system effectors required to achieve the goal. Consequently, a feedforward movement plan initiated in the guided system by a spatial specification of the goal received from the guiding system will deviate from the targeted location by the amount of the misalignment.

We assume that the subordinate guided system together with effectors and sensors of the superordinate guiding system constitute what is called the controlled system in control systems theory. The spatially coded control signals from the guiding system controller are used both to control its own effectors and to specify the behavioral goal for the guided system. Feedback from the guided system is available to the guiding system only through its own exteroceptor. Sensors (extero-ceptors and proprioceptors) of the guided system only serve the controller of the guided system, which may operate autonomously to achieve the goal specified by the guiding system. The case in which remote sensors of one sensorimotor system provide information to another sensorimotor system constitutes a reversal in the direction of guidance between the two systems. The only direct exchange of spatial information between systems is through spatially coded control signals.

Feedback Compensation

If online feedback is available to a controller, unexpected deviation from an ongoing feedforward movement plan (i.e., error) can be detected and the spatial difference between actual outcome and required outcome can be used under feedback control to reduce or eliminate performance error (see Figs. 5.2 and 3.3). In a sensorimotor system, feedback is normally available from both exteroceptors and proprioceptors. However, when separate sensorimotor systems are coordinatively linked, the flow of control (and information) is from guiding system to guided system. The guiding system has direct access only to its own sensors, not those of the guided system. The directionality of guidance linkages places constraints on how feedback can be used to compensate for performance errors arising from spatial misalignment of sensorimotor systems.

For example, in the common case of *visual guidance* of the limb, a goal specification from higher centers together with sensory input about the current state of the task–work space (both exteroceptive information about the content of visual space and proprioceptive information about present position of the eyes) is used to select a feedforward movement plan for achieving the targeted position. The movement plan includes specification of both an initiating to-be-achieved target position and expected intermediate positions in the movement path. These spatial specifications provide the basis for both monitoring sensory input for predictable disturbances (feedforward control) and providing a continuous reference for detecting errors (feedback control). The control signals associated with these spatial specifications are used by the eye–head (visual) sensorimotor system to control its own effectors and are sent to the hand–shoulder (proprioceptive) sensorimotor system as a goal specification for this guided system.

Control signals are, therefore, assumed to be spatially coded commands that can serve for goal specification. Having received these instructions, the control structures, sensors, and effectors in the hand–shoulder system can operate autonomously toward the targeted position in proprioceptive limb space. That is, the received goal specification selects a feedforward movement plan in the guided system that can be executed without further input from the guiding system.

However, when visual (exteroceptor) input is distorted, for example, by laterally displacing prisms, instructions to the hand–shoulder system produce limb (effector) locations in proprioceptive space that differ from corresponding locations in visual space by the amount of the prismatically induced spatial misalignment of the sensorimotor systems. The consequent unexpected deviations of the limb from the movement plan (i.e., errors) can be detected by the visual exteroceptor. The spatial difference (vector) between planned and actual limb locations can be added to the control signal from the eye–head system to produce an online correction in limb movement. That is, the spatial difference between actual outcome (positioning of the guided system sensed by the visual exteroceptor) and required outcome (the reference given by the goal specification from the visual system) can be used by the local controller of the guided system to force its effector toward the target. In this manner, performance error can be reduced or eliminated.

Note that the operation of the eye–head system is unaffected by the distortion; optical displacement affects corresponding locations between visual and proprioceptive limb space but not relative location in visual space.[3] Note also that prismatically induced error is not detected by the guided hand–shoulder system; it is simply doing what it has been told to do. In the absence of a local error source (e.g., an unexpected load imposed on the limb) the selected movement plan in the guided system may be executed flawlessly. Still, the location achieved in limb space will not match the targeted location in visual space. Lacking exteroceptor access to the behavior of the visual system, the hand–shoulder system cannot detect the error made by the visual system.

In the case just discussed, detection of the prismatically induced error and computation of the necessary correction occurs in the guiding visual system, whereas execution of the correction is done by the guided hand–shoulder system. The situation is somewhat different when the direction of guidance between eyes and hand is reversed. In the case of *proprioceptive guidance,* error detection, and

---

[3] This is not true for prisms placed on the eye itself (e.g., via contact lenses) rather than in front of the eyes (e.g., via goggles). We discuss this case in chapter 6 under the heading "Intrasystem Misalignment."

correction computation cannot occur in the guiding hand–shoulder system because this sensorimotor system lacks exteroceptor access to the visual system. Instead, feedback compensation occurs entirely in the guided visual system.

To look at the initially nonvisible hand, the eye–head system first receives goal-specifying control signals from the hand–shoulder system. Local execution of the selected feedforward movement plan in the visual system fails to achieve fixation of the target because the goal specification received from the hand–shoulder system does not pick out the corresponding locations in visual space when the two sensorimotor system are spatially misaligned. However, the visual exteroceptor can detect the discrepancy between achieved (fixated) location and required goal location. This spatial error can be used locally to execute a corrective saccade. The visual system knows what the hand looks like and recognizes when the goal of fixation is not achieved.[4] Autonomy of sensorimotor systems includes access to (higher order) pattern information that can be utilized for goal specification in addition to remote guidance signals. As a further example, the hand has access to information about the shape of a cup and can distinguish when it has grasped a saucer instead.

A similar account of feedback compensation applies to the coordinative linkage of eye–head visual and foot–hip locomotion systems and can be developed for coordinative linkages with the ear–neck system illustrated in Fig. 5.1. For auditory guidance (by the ear–neck system) of proprioceptive (hand–shoulder) or locomotion (foot–hip) systems with spatial misalignment (e.g., pseudophonic displacement), the sound shadow of a doorway may initiate limb movement and the audible impact of the guided system (hand or foot striking the door frame) may serve for error detection in the guiding auditory system and computation of a corrective feedback control signal sent to the guided system. Similarly, the sound made by a moving limb (footfall or the arm sliding along a rough surface) may serve as corrective feedback for an orienting response of the auditory system that was initiated by spatially coded control signals from the limb itself (i.e., proprioceptive guidance).

When a target is both visible and audible, feedback compensation may originate from either the visual (eye–head) system or the auditory (ear–neck) system when these systems are coordinatively linked (not shown directly in Fig. 5.1), depending on which system is serving the guiding role. When neither (none) of the coordinately linked sensorimotor system has exteroceptor access to the other(s) (e.g., the possible linkage of foot–hip and hand–shoulder systems in Fig. 5.1), online feedback compensation may not be possible. In the next section, we consider how performance error may nevertheless be reduced by offline compensation based on knowledge of results.

Feedback control strategies that normally serve to correct ordinary performance errors such as those arising from imprecise encoding of spatial position, imprecise execution of a movement command, or unexpected external disturbances can be

---

[4]Note that such pattern recognition is also necessary for feedback compensation in visual guidance. The visual system must know what the hand and target look like to recognize an error.

recruited to correct for performance errors arising from spatial misalignment of sensorimotor systems. However, such feedback compensation does not require realignment of the sensorimotor systems.

In all of the preceding illustrations, feedback compensation was achieved in spite of the fact that, in objective terms, the coordinated systems operated with different spatial coordinates for the same spatial position. Indeed, feedback compensation depends on the misalignment; without the misalignment, feedback compensation would not be needed. Online feedback error correction may produce adaptive performance but does not remove the misalignment (see also Fig. 4.3). In chapter 6, however, we show how feedback compensation via difference codes may leave the initial position movement code unchanged, thereby establishing conditions for misalignment detection and consequent realignment.

Knowledge of Results Compensation

If offline knowledge of results is available to a controller after an action is completed, the spatial difference between endpoint effector position and targeted position can be used to change (by the amount of terminal error) the goal specification that initiates feedforward control, selecting a (perhaps slightly) different movement plan such that performance error is reduced or eliminated for the next action (see Figs. 5.2 and 3.3). Within a sensorimotor system, knowledge of results is normally available from both exteroceptors and proprioceptors, as well as from augmenting sources (e.g., verbal feedback). As with online feedback, offline knowledge of results from sensors in the guided sensorimotor system is not available to the guiding system. Availability of such sensory information can only be accomplished by reversing the coordinative linkage, changing the guiding and guided roles of the sensorimotor systems. However, augmented knowledge of results may be available to correct performance error locally in the guided system.

As a first illustration, consider visual guidance of the limb in which terminal error for the guided (hand–shoulder or leg–hip) system may be available to the guiding visual system via its own exteroceptor (or augmenting sources of information). Such knowledge of results can be used to select a different spatially specified goal for the next action. This amended goal specification is sent by the guiding system to its own effectors and to the guided system where it is used to select a movement plan that better achieves the targeted position. Such knowledge of results compensation normally serves to correct for inaccurate encoding in the guiding system of a target's spatial position. However, it can also be used to correct performance error arising from spatial misalignment of sensorimotor systems.

When visual (exteroceptor) input is distorted, for example, by laterally displacing prisms, instructions to the hand–shoulder system produces an endpoint location for the hand that differs from the targeted location by the amount and direction of the prismatic displacement when online feedback compensation is absent or by some lesser amount when feedback compensation is incomplete. The terminal error (sensed visually or by augmented information) is used to specify a virtual target located to the side of the actual target by the amount and direction of the terminal error, such that on receipt and execution of these instructions, the guided limb better achieves the target with the next action. In this manner, performance error can be reduced or eliminated over successive actions.

Although terminal error could provide a measure of spatial misalignment of sensorimotor systems (especially in the absence of feedback compensation), it is not used in this manner in knowledge of results compensation. No explicit comparison is made between achieved position in limb space and targeted position in visual space. Rather, the comparison is between positions in visual space and the difference is used to reset the goal specification for the guided system. The knowledge of results compensation process is the same as is employed when the target physically changes it position over successive actions; a new target is specified for each action. The same process cannot be used to detect both changes in the world and changes in internal function (see chapter 3).

With proprioceptive guidance of the visual system (e.g., by hand–shoulder or leg–hip systems), terminal error detected by the visual exteroceptor can be used to associate a local goal specification with the remote guidance signal so as to achieve the targeted position with the next action. Not illustrated in Fig. 5.3 is the short-term memory capacity of sensorimotor systems necessary to store the correction derived from knowledge of results until the next action can be initiated. In the next section we consider how, with extended practice, this short-term association can be developed to form a more persistent correction contingent upon situational cues provided by prism exposure.

Similar accounts of performance correction over successive actions apply for auditory guidance (by the ear–head system) of proprioceptive (hand–shoulder) and locomotion (leg–hip) systems under pseudophonic displacement. Auditory information (action-contingent sounds) about the terminal error (knowledge of results) produced by an action can be used to select a different movement plan with a different initiating target location in the guided or guiding ear–head system such that the next action can more closely achieve the targeted location. When visual and auditory systems are coordinatively linked, knowledge of results compensation for performance error arising from prismatic or pseudophonic misalignment (or both) can be achieved over successive actions by selecting compensatory movement plans in either the visual or auditory system, depending on the direction of guidance required by a specific task.

Knowledge of results does not depend exclusively upon exteroceptor function. Because of this, it can be used to correct performance errors arising from misalignment of sensorimotor systems that lack exteroceptor access to each others performance. For example, touching a door frame with the hand may initiate locomotion to orient on a doorway. Subsequent contact of the hand with the opposite side of the door frame can be used to select a different movement plan for the locomotion system to more accurately orient on the doorway. We know of no experimental examples of misalignment between hand–shoulder and leg–hip sensorimotor systems. Pathology might produce such misalignment, and knowledge of results eventually could be used to achieve movement through, for example, a doorway. Moreover, augmented knowledge of results through verbal feedback might enable selection of a compensatory feedforward movement plan.

Knowledge of results can be available after an action is completed, either through exteroceptor function or augmenting information sources. In this case, the goal specification can be amended by using the amount of terminal error to select a feedforward movement plan that succeeds, or nearly succeeds, in achieving the target. Such offline compensation for terminal error may be an alternative to online error correction if feedback is not available or it may operate in addition to feedback error correction. Again, however, note that misalignment of coordinated sensorimotor systems remains, even though performance may be adaptive. The guided system may achieve the secondary targeted location, but the spatial representation of the original primary target in the guiding system remains different (in objective terms) from the target representation in the guided system. Indeed, the spatial representations must remain unchanged if the relative difference between actual and virtual targets is to be a reliable means of achieving the target. Thus, offline use of knowledge of results can interfere with realignment in much the same way it can interfere with motor learning by failing to activate the to-be-learning motor organization (Lee, White, & Carnahan, 1990; Salmoni, Schmidt, & Walter, 1984).

Associative Learning

If information is available that discriminates a condition of spatial misalignment between coordinatively linked sensorimotor systems and if extended practice on the coordination task is provided, short-term knowledge of results compensation can be developed into a more persistent strategy for improving performance that can be deployed quickly whenever the condition of misalignment is detected. Such learning normally strengthens the associative linkage between input (initial conditions and predictable disturbances) and output (control signals) of a feedforward controller to produce a task-specific movement plan (see Figs. 5.2 and 3.3), but can also serve to develop a compensatory feedforward movement plan contingently activated by a condition of misalignment. Indeed, there is some evidence for such contingent prism adaptation (Bingham, Muchisky, & Romack, 1991; Bridgeman, Anand, Browman, & Welch, 1992; McGonigle & Flook, 1978; Romack, Buss, & Bingham, 1992; Welch, Bridgeman, Anand, & Browman, 1991, 1993).

For example, with visual guidance of the limb, several sources of information are available that enable the actor to discriminate presence or absence of prismatic displacement. These include the prism-bearing goggles that the actor wears (Kravitz, 1972; Welch, 1971a), the small color and shape distortions that usually accompany prismatic displacement (Welch, 1978), and verbal or nonverbal information that a change in the prisms has been made. These cues may become associated with the virtual displacement that terminal error (knowledge of results) indicates can be used to select a movement plan in the visual system controller that achieves the actual targeted position.

With extended practice, the associative linkage becomes strengthened to the point that the compensatory feedforward movement plan is activated whenever the various cues indicate the presence of the misalignment. In this manner, whenever the misalignment is reintroduced, performance may be error-free, or nearly so, even at the onset of the misalignment.

Moreover, because ancillary sensory information (e.g., color and shape distortions) can indicate the direction of prismatic displacement, contingent movement plans can be learned for different prismatic displacements and a learned movement plan may partially transfer to a new displacement. In general, contingent movement plans may transfer (generalize) to other misalignment conditions depending on the similarity between the novel misalignment condition and the condition under which the original plan was learned. Distinct contingencies can be learned if misalignment conditions are discriminably different.

Similar compensation by associative learning can occur for the various directional guidance linkages illustrated in Fig. 5.1, when knowledge of results and misalignment-contingent information are available. However, like knowledge of results compensation, associative learning compensates for, but does not remove, the misalignment. Indeed, both knowledge of results and associative learning compensation are antithetical to realignment. They remove the possible basis for misalignment detection. That is, the spatial coordinates of the actual target in the guiding system are *replaced* by spatial coordinates in the guided system that achieve the target. There can be, therefore, no comparison of corresponding spatial positions for the coordinately linked sensorimotor systems and no possibility of detecting the misalignment. Moreover, such associative learning appears to be fundamentally different from the kind of learning involved in spatial realignment (Bedford, 1993a, 1993b; see also chapter 3).

SUMMARY

The adaptive processes that serve everyday perceptual–motor coordination can be recruited to compensate for performance errors produced by misalignment between spatial representations. However, coordination is exclusively concerned with the exchange of control signals between sensorimotor systems. Because purely sensory signals are not exchanged, misalignment between sensorimotor spatial representations cannot be detected or realignment initiated by such ordinary adaptive processes.

Resetting the movement plan goal based on knowledge of results or learning a movement plan contingent on the misalignment can produce adaptive performance. Such knowledge of results compensation and associative learning precludes misalignment detection because the distorted, error-producing spatial control signal is replaced with an error-reducing signal.

Feedback compensation may, however, establish conditions for misalignment detection and consequent realignment. In this case, the error-corrective, difference code remains distinct from the position code that initiated movement.

Chapter 6

ALIGNMENT
AND REALIGNMENT

In chapter 5 we developed a model of perceptual–motor coordination in which misalignment-induced performance errors can be corrected. Such adaptive performance does not address the more fundamental problem of spatial misalignment among sensorimotor systems. Strategic (feedforward and feedback) control and associative (motor) learning are realized by the exchange of control signals among sensorimotor structures that can compensate for performance error induced by spatial misalignment. These adaptive processes do not require the comparison of corresponding positions among spatial representations that is necessary for the detection of misalignment and consequent realignment.

In the present chapter, we extend the model to account for spatial alignment and realignment. We begin by articulating the internal structure and function of sensorimotor systems that we believe is responsible for spatial mapping among internal representations. Then, we specify the encoding and decoding operations that enable communication among the various sensorimotor spatial representations via mediating noetic space. In the third section, we show how encoding and decoding parameters are supplied to enable task-specific calibration of spatially aligned sensorimotor representations. Finally, we show how, under conditions of feedback error-correction, misalignment can be detected and realignment initiated, with illustrations for both intrasystem and intersystem misalignment.

SENSORIMOTOR SYSTEMS

Figure 6.1 represents the assumed internal structure of a sensorimotor system. Strategic control and associative learning are functions of the *controller*, which may operate autonomously or respond to remote guidance signals from another sensorimotor system. For simplicity, feedforward and feedback functions are collapsed into a single controller, and the two kinds of control with their distinctive control signals are only implicit in this figure. A controller sends control signals (*efference*), which are spatial codes for desired positions, to its associated effector, and receives spatial information about position in personal space (*proprioceptor*) and extrapersonal space (*exteroceptor*). The broken line input to the controller illustrates the

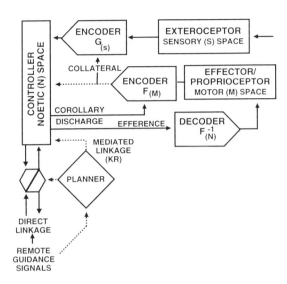

FIG. 6.1.   Internal structure and function of sensorimotor systems. Strategic control is the function of
the (feedforward and feedback) controller, that may operate autonomously or under remote guidance.
General transformational operators embedded in encoders map positions in sensory (**S**) space or motor
(**M**) space onto common noetic (**N**) space, whereas inverse transformation maps noetically coded
commands onto motor space. Calibration signals (collateral and corollary discharge) enable noetic
representation of present spatial relationship among sensorimotor elements.

assumption that, although proprioceptor and exteroceptor normally provide the
same information about spatial position, a controller favors the sensory (exteroceptor) signal (McCloskey, 1981) when it is available, because of the additional
information provided in this spatially extended input.

Remote online control signals (feedback and feedforward) are represented as
direct linkage, in which the control signals used by a controller in a remote guiding
sensorimotor system are also used to direct a local guided controller. Offline control
signals derived from knowledge of results (KR) are represented as *mediated
linkage*, reflecting the larger planner involvement in the utilization of information
that must be retained over successive movements and that may not be expressed
directly in terms of control signals (e.g., augmented or verbal feedback). In the next
two sections, we first develop the spatial mapping function of encoding–decoding
operations and then show how task-specific calibration can be established among
spatially aligned sensorimotor representations.

ALIGNMENT (SPATIAL MAPPING)

Spatial mapping is the function of *encoder* and *decoder* operators within a sensorimotor system. The spatial representations for the *sensory space* (**S**) of an extero-

ceptor and the *motor space*[1] (**M**) of an effector with its associated sensor (proprio-ceptor) are distinct from each other and from the spatial representations of other sensorimotor systems. Communication between exteroceptors and effector–pro-prioceptors in a sensorimotor system and between sensorimotor systems is medi-ated by *noetic space* (**N**), a spatial representation common to all sensorimotor systems. Encoders contain unique *transformational operators* (see chapter 2),[2] that translate between motor space ($F_{(M)}$) or sensory space ($G_{(s)}$) and noetic space. Decoders contain an inverse operator ($F_{(N)}^{-1}$) that transforms coordinates in noetic space into coordinates in motor space. Because the exteroceptor does not have a motor function, there is no inverse operator. Alignment among sensory and motor spatial representations in a sensorimotor system and between the various sensorimotor systems is established by encoding and decoding operations via mediating noetic space.

A single spatial representation common to all parts of the perceptual–motor system would seem to have several advantages over other ways of solving the sensorimotor mapping problem.[3] There could be unique mappings between every possible combination of sensory and motor systems, but the number and complexity of such mappings would seem prohibitive. Moreover, central programming of motor behavior would be difficult, if possible at all, in such a case. Each movement program would have to be tailored to the unique spatial translation requirements of the systems involved. In contrast, noetic space permits central programming of movements by general commands that can be transformed into coordinates of a specific sensorimotor system. Sensorimotor systems can then be strategically organized to meet changing task demands.

The mediational role of noetic space means that it is self-centered rather than object-centered. The primitive function of noetic space is communication among the many unique sensory and motor spaces so that perceptual–motor coordination can be achieved. Self-centered representation is consistent with our phenomenal sense of perceptual–motor space and would seem to be the most efficient solution to the fundamental problem of sensorimotor mapping. Noetic space should be considered as different from object-centered representations that mediate object recognition (Biederman, 1985, 1987). This distinction is similar to the dissociation of brain functions serving pattern recognition and motor behavior.[4]

Moreover, we assume noetic space to be a hierarchical representation in the sense that some parts are represented relative to other parts. The reference point can be shifted depending on the task (see also, Generalization 3, chapter 4). For example, in

---

[1]Here, and in all that follows, we intend *motor space* to denote kinematic frames that represent movement in terms that the perceptual system can understand. Dynamic frames that represent movement in terms of forces are another level of description that is outside the domain of the present concern. (See also chapter 2).

[2]For additional discussion of transformational operators, see Churchland (1986), Dodwell (1970), Pellionisz and Llinás (1985), and Soechting (1989).

[3]The idea of a common space has long been implicit in psychological research (for reviews, see Auerbach & Sperling, 1974; Fisher, 1962a, 1962b, 1968) and recently was expressed explicitly (Grossberg & Kuperstein, 1989; Howard, 1982; Jackendoff & Landau, 1994).

[4]Recent discussions of this dissociation can be found in Jeannerod (1994), Milner and Goodale (1993), and Mishkin (1993).

reaching for visible objects, the arm and upper body might be represented as a functional superordinate unit referenced on the head, a hand–head system. At the planning level, terminal head-centric coordinates might be set in noetic space by the eye–head system. These target coordinates could then be realized, kinematically and dynamically, by subcomponents synergistically constrained to act as a unit. For purposes requiring finer manipulation, like writing, the functional unit of organization might be fingers to elbow or shoulders. Thus, the proposed hierarchical nature of noetic representation enables task-specific, strategic organization of subsystems into functional superordinate systems, perhaps simply by changing the reference point in noetic space.

One especially remarkable virtue of transformational operators should be noted: Because they are general transforms, the noetic representation they produce is not restricted to the sensorimotor space that is the source of their input. Noetic space can be extrapolated beyond the limits of a particular sensorimotor space. Thus, transformational operators form the basis for extended noetic space, a space in which higher level processes can move independently of body movements or sensory limitations. The general nature of transformational operators is most dramatically demonstrated by the fact that impossible limb positions are extrapolated when effector movement is prevented, but continued changes in muscle afference are induced by artificial means (Craske, 1977; McCloskey, 1973).

CALIBRATION

We distinguish calibration from alignment. *Calibration* is the representation of the present relationship in noetic space among various sensorimotor elements in preparation for an action. Calibration, therefore, establishes the present condition of the task–work space in noetic terms and permits movement planning and evaluation. *Alignment* is the long-term, steady-state relationship among sensorimotor elements by virtue of which corresponding positions in the various sensorimotor representations map onto common positions in noetic space. Alignment is a prerequisite for calibration. Unless transformational operators align sensorimotor representations, calibration will fail to veridically represent the relationship among sensorimotor elements. In this section, we discuss calibration, assuming alignment. In the next section we illustrate how alignment is established.

The *collateral* and *corollary discharge* shown in Fig. 6.1 are calibration signals that enable noetic representation of the present relationship among sensory and motor frames. These signals specify the present noetic values for the origin location and axes orientation of a sensory or motor frame. These values serve as input to the transformational operator that maps positions in sensory or motor space onto corresponding positions in noetic space. Given the position (origin location and axes orientation) of a sensory or motor frame in noetic coordinates, then all positions in sensory or motor space can be transformed into corresponding positions in noetic space.

For example, the collateral of present eye position in noetic space specifies the position of the retinal frame in noetic coordinates and enables transformation of all retinal positions into noetic positions. Similarly, a collateral of present position for a limb segment specifies the position of a tactile frame in noetic coordinates and enables transformation of all tactile positions into noetic positions. And, a collateral of present head position specifies the position of the auditory frame in noetic coordinates and enables transformation of all auditory positions into noetic positions.

We make the parsimonious assumption that the foregoing description applies to all sensorimotor systems, that these primitive units of perceptual–motor organization have similar internal structure and function. Such an assumption may be most controversial with regards to the eye–head system, in which the position sense is frequently assumed to be solely a corollary discharge function (outflow theory; Helmholtz, 1909/1962) without proprioceptor input (inflow theory; Sherrington, 1918). However, recent work demonstrates a proprioceptive basis for eye position (Matin, Stevens, & Picoult, 1983; Skavenski, 1972; Skavenski et al., 1972). There now seems sufficient grounds for assuming a cooperative inflow–outflow basis for the visual position sense as well as for other position senses like that for a limb (see also McCloskey, 1981).

For example, the corollary discharge of an eye movement command expresses the present position (origin location and axes orientation) of the motor frame for the eye muscles in noetic coordinates. Such information is necessary to enable the inverse transformation of noetically coded (body-centric) commands into coordinates that the head-centric motor system can interpret. We assume that the same information is also used to transform positions in motor space into positions in noetic space. In a sense, the encoder and decoder operators for the effector–proprioceptor unit shown in Fig. 6.1 are not distinct mechanisms but represent the different directions of transformation. Thus, corollary discharge is indirectly implicated in the visual position sense in that it is involved in producing the collateral calibration signal. Note also that because the corollary discharge is distinct from the motor command (efference), mapping of effector position onto noetic space can be maintained by continuous activation of the corollary discharge when there is no overt movement of the effector (e.g., no eye movement).

In general, we assume that the corollary discharge of a motor command to an effector segment specifies the endpoint position of a more proximal segment in noetic space and, therefore, the noetic position of the motor frame for the more distal controlled segment. Figure 6.2 illustrates this cascade of calibration signals for a multisegment effector. The encoded position for a proximal segment provides calibration that enables both encoding and decoding operators for the next distal segment. Ultimately, the cascade originates from a body-centric frame, thereby assuring calibration of segments in noetic space.

For example, when movement is confined to the limb, shoulder position provides the body-centric parameters for encoding and decoding operations for the upper limb. The upper limb then provides calibration for the lower limb, and the position of the lower limb endpoint (wrist) in turn specifies the noetic position (origin location and axes orientation) of the motor frame for the hand. The cascade

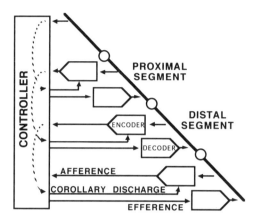

FIG. 6.2. Cascade of calibration signals. In a multisegment effector, the corollary discharge of a motor command to an effector segment specifies the endpoint position of a more proximal segment in noetic space and, therefore, the noetic position of the motor frame for the more distal, controlled segment.

is similarly developed for the proximal-to-distal segments of the hand. For simplicity, exteroceptor functions have not been included in Fig. 6.2, but when exteroceptor signals are available (e.g., from tactile surfaces of the various limb segments), they may also contribute to calibration, as illustrated in Fig. 6.1.

Note also that calibration is not restricted to local signals in a sensorimotor system. The observation that target pointing accuracy improves when the hand is seen shortly before movement initiation (Jeannerod, 1988, 1991a; Jeannerod & Prablanc, 1983; Prablanc, Echallier, Jeannerod et al., 1979), especially when the hand is seen during movement preparation (Elliott, 1988; Elliott, Carson, Goodman, & Chua, 1991; Rossetti, Stelmach, Desmurget, Prablanc, & Jeannerod, 1994), is evidence that calibration signals may originate in a remote, guiding sensorimotor system.

The perception–action cascade provides the necessary control elements for strategic perceptual–motor performance outlined in chapters 1 and 5. Although the various effector segments are structurally serial, motor control (efference) and calibration (corollary discharge) occur in parallel for all of the segments. A movement plan can specify desired positions synergistically for all segments of an effector. Feedforward control can predictively compensate for an anticipated perturbation in the movement of one segment by adjustment in the movement of another segment. Indeed, movement plans and feedforward control can exist for strategically selected segment configurations when freedom of movement is constrained, for example, to the lower limb. Overt errors can be detected and corrected online by feedback control. Of course, knowledge of results can be used offline to modify the movement plan.

In the assumed functions of the collateral and corollary discharge, we follow the suggestion (Matthews, 1977; McCloskey, 1981) that such signals are necessary to disambiguate afferent signals. We further adopt the position (MacKay, 1973; MacKay & Mittelstaedt, 1974) that these signals serve an interpretive (e.g., corollary discharge) function rather than a cancellation (efferent copy) function (McCloskey, 1981).[5] The function of these signals is *not* to create a stable world by subtracting out effector movement. Stability is an assumed quality of noetic representation, the stored map of the environment.

For instance, movement of the retina or the tactile surface of the palm over an unchanging stimulus field is analogous to moving a transparent overlay across a map of a well-known neighborhood. The position of the overlay is specified in the framework of the continuously available neighborhood map, not the other way around. The overlay serves only to highlight (e.g., foveate or touch) portions of the neighborhood. The map is not continuously built up from successive overlay positions. Change in the neighborhood (i.e., object movement), however, is recorded by altering the noetic coordinates of the affected content in the neighborhood map. This memorial function is not illustrated in the present figures.

Note also that performance evaluation is not a function of the encoding operators. These operators provide necessary information, but predictive feedforward control and error-corrective feedback control are functions of the combined controller in Fig. 6.1. Encoders (and the inverse decoder) only function to establish spatial alignment between sensory and motor space, and because this alignment is mediated by noetic space, it also serves to align the various sensorimotor systems. In the next section, we show how, when feedback is available, evidence of spatial misalignment between sensory and motor space (intrasystem discordance) and between sensorimotor systems (intersystem discordance) can be derived from collateral and corollary discharge information to motivate realignment.

REALIGNMENT (ADAPTIVE ENCODERS)

Prismatic distortions, as well as natural processes of growth, pathology, and drift, produce situations where representations in sensory and motor frames of the same position in the task–work space do *not* transform into the same position in noetic space. We believe detection of such misalignment and consequent realignment is a function of encoding operations. Briefly, *realignment* is a long-term parametric adjustment of transformational operators, in contrast to *calibration,* which changes for different tasks.[6] However, detection of misalignment and consequent realignment is critically dependent upon goal-directed action by the sensorimotor system in which the encoders are embedded. We first sketch the adaptive function of encoders in general terms. In subsequent sections, we show how realignment can occur in exteroceptor or proprioceptor encoders, depending on the action of an isolated sensorimotor system (intrasystem realignment), and how the locus of

---

[5]See also Abbs et al. (1984), Bullock and Grossberg (1988), and Szentágothai and Arbib (1975).

[6]The distinction between calibration and realignment is analogous to the difference between calibrating an instrument for a particular task and selecting another measuring instrument that also must be calibrated for each task.

realignment depends on the direction of guidance between coordinated sensorimotor systems (intersystem realignment).

Figure 6.3 illustrates the assumed internal structure and function of an adaptive encoder. Misalignment detection is enabled by comparison of the calibration signal with the output of the transformational operator $T_{(A)}$. The calibration signal specifies the origin location and axes orientation of a sensory or motor frame in noetic space. When the sensorimotor system, in which the encoder is embedded, orients to a target (i.e., the sensory or motor frame is centered on the target), the noetically coded target position should ordinarily match the noetically coded calibration signal in a spatially aligned system. With goal-directed action, a calibration signal acquires the role of expected position and output of the transformational operator signals the achieved position. In a system whose sensory and motor spaces are misaligned, however, expected and achieved positions will not match and the discrepancy $N - T_{(A)}$ (discordance) signals a gradual adjustment in the parameters of the transformational operator. This parametric adjustment is permanent (until a new misalignment occurs), such that the same calibration signal will now produce a veridical mapping of sensory or motor space onto noetic space. Because sensory and motor space are realigned with noetic space, they are realigned with each other.

Marshaling the various resources of a sensorimotor system to orient on a target is the mechanistic implementation of the common action solution to the correspondence problem discussed in chapter 3. Concerted action by the various elements of a sensorimotor system produces synchronous spatial representations that can be compared to detect internal errors. Ordinary performance errors are filtered out by

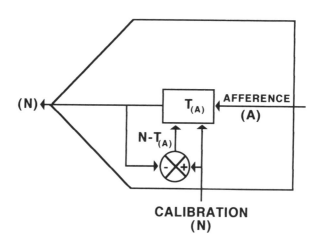

FIG. 6.3. Internal structure and function of adaptive encoders. Coordination of spatially misaligned sensorimotor elements produces discordance $(N - T_{(A)})$ between position expected from calibration signals (collateral or corollary discharge) and achieved position encoded by the transformational operator $(T_{(A)})$. This discordance initiates a long response time, incremental change in parameters of the transformational operator to restore alignment between afference (A) signals from sensory or motor space and noetic (N) space.

predictive feedforward control or by online feedback control. Moreover, we assume that ordinary performance errors that arise from imprecision in sensorimotor operations are randomly distributed, in contrast to performance errors arising from misalignment that are consistent in direction.

Because the most common natural source of misalignment (drift) produces slowly developing misalignments of small magnitudes, evolution has produced an adaptive mechanism that has a long response time and which makes only incremental adjustments. Consequently, any discordance produced by imprecision in orienting to a target will signal only a slow, small change in parameters of the transformational operator and such random discordance will average out in the ordinary operation of spatially aligned sensorimotor elements. Only the consistent discordance produced by misalignment will produce any substantial, cumulative change in transformation parameters.

Goal-directed action is one requirement for misalignment detection and consequent realignment. To the extent that coordination requires intentional processes and the limited capacity for such processing is not available, goal-directed action and consequent misalignment detection and reduction will not occur (Generalization 5, chapter 4). Another requirement is the availability of exteroceptor feedback. Without exteroceptor input, there can be no achieved target position output of the transformational operator for comparison with the expected target position (collateral). We assume that without such input, the comparator cannot operate. No discordance signal will be produced, and no realignment of sensory space will occur.

Moreover, without exteroceptor feedback, there can be no discordance in the proprioceptor encoder. Given an initiating target position, an effector will move to orient on that position, the encoded achieved target position will match the expected target position (corollary discharge), and the misalignment between sensory and motor space will not be detected. A feedforward movement plan can be executed flawlessly and proprioceptor feedback will indicate target achievement. Only the exteroceptor can provide the error signal (difference code) necessary to drive the *relative* position of the effector toward the target position.

Only feedback from an exteroceptor with an extended field can provide the needed kind of error signal. We assume that such feedback control leaves unchanged the corollary discharge input (position code) to the proprioceptor encoder. To perform its calibration function, the corollary discharge must code the *absolute* position of the motor frame in noetic space. Thus, feedback control can establish conditions in which achieved effector position does not match the expected effector position, enabling misalignment detection and realignment of motor space.

Error-free performance is necessary for maximal realignment of motor space. To the extent that a targeted position is not achieved, the motor frame will not be centered on the target and discordance will underestimate the needed realignment. On the other hand, error-free performance removes the stimulus for realignment of sensory space. When the effector achieves the targeted position under feedback control, thereby removing the performance error induced by the misalignment, the collateral input to the exteroceptor encoder signals a noetic position for the sensory frame that matches the noetically coded position of the target in sensory space. To the extent that performance is not error free, some stimulus remains for cooperative realignment of both sensory and motor space.

Offline correction of performance using knowledge of results disables misalignment detection and consequent realignment of both sensory and motor space. When a virtual target is selected to correct a previous performance error produced by misalignment, the effector orients on that virtual target and the achieved position matches the expected position in the proprioceptor encoder. No discordance is registered. Moreover, the actual target will now be centered in the sensory frame and no discordance signal will be present in the exteroceptor encoder. Thus, the direct linkage shown in Fig. 6.1 is necessary for detection of misalignment between sensorimotor systems and consequent realignment. Mediated linkage precludes misalignment detection and realignment.

Misalignment can occur either in a sensorimotor system (intrasystem), with discordance between exteroceptor and proprioceptor functions, or between sensorimotor systems (intersystem), in which the discordance is described as between systems. In either case, the locus of parametric adjustment in transformational operators depends on the manner in which sensorimotor elements are coordinated. We now illustrate these two cases with examples from prism adaptation. We refer to Figs. 6.1 and 6.3 in the following discussion of intrasystem and intersystem misalignment.

Intrasystem Misalignment

An experimental example of intrasystem discordance is the case where a wedge prism is mounted directly on the eye via a contact lens and subjects are required to follow contours with their eye (Festinger, Burnham, Ono, & Bamber, 1967; Slotnick, 1969). The apparent curvature produced by such prisms will cause misalignment between eye positions (proprioceptor function) necessary to achieve a target and target positions on the retina (exteroceptor function).

Initially, the eyes (effector) will achieve a target position indicated by encoded retinal position, within precision limits of the system, and there will be no discrepancy between encoded and expected (corollary discharge) effector position. However, position encoded by the exteroceptor will differ from the expected (collateral) target position. The eyes may move to the commanded position, but the target will not be foveated. Phenomenally, the contour appears to move, avoiding the eyes. This discordance between expected and achieved positions should prompt realignment of the exteroceptor transformation ($G_{(s)}$ in Fig. 6.1) to agreement with the proprioceptor transformation ($F_{(M)}$ in Fig. 6.1); a realignment of sensory space.

However, visual feedback (i.e., the error between target and fovea) may prompt a difference movement command from the controller to the effector to zero-out the error. Such error correction may remove the motive (discordance) for exteroceptor realignment, but should leave unchanged the expected (corollary discharge) effector position. (Recall that the calibration function of the corollary discharge requires that it be a position code, not a difference code). The eye will move to foveate the target, but the expected eye position will be different from the achieved eye position. The resultant discordance should prompt realignment of the proprioceptor transformation ($F_{(M)}$ in Fig. 6.1) to agreement with the exteroceptor transformation ($G_{(s)}$ in Fig. 6.1); a realignment of motor space.

Thus, in the case where the anomaly occurs in sensory (exteroceptor) space, realignment will occur in exteroceptor or proprioceptor encoders depending on whether position or difference movement codes are sent to the effector. The observation that curvature adaptation is greater for saccadic eye movements (position commands) than for tracking eye movements (difference commands) suggests that exteroceptor realignment may be the more rapid process (Festinger et al., 1967; Slotnick, 1969).

We are not aware of any experimental instances of anomalies in motor space. In the present theoretical framework, anomalies could arise in effector or proprioceptor functions. In the first case, the effector would fail to achieve the commanded position, and in the second case, proprioceptive sensors would fail to veridically represent the achieved position. In either case, the encoded achieved position would not match the expected position (corollary discharge), with consequent discordance in the proprioceptor encoder and parametric adjustment of its transformational operator ($F_{(M)}$ in Fig. 6.1). However, if exteroceptor feedback is used to force the effector to the target position, the locus of discordance would be shifted to the exteroceptor encoder with consequent parametric adjustment of this transformational operator ($G_{(s)}$ in Fig. 6.1). Thus, when the source of anomaly is motor space, the effect of feedback correction on the locus of realignment should be opposite that occurring when the anomaly arises from sensory space.

The locus of intrasystem discordance and realignment depends on visual feedback availability and utilization whether the source of the misalignment is in visual or motor space. Because the amount of adaptive change in any encoder at any time is only a fraction of that needed, there will be remaining motivation for realignment in the other encoder until the total discordance is removed and realignment of sensory and motor spaces is achieved. Note, however, that offline use of knowledge of results in a sensorimotor system may limit realignment. We discuss this and other limitations on realignment in chapter 7.

A similar illustration might be developed for intrasystem misalignment in nonvisual sensorimotor systems like the hand–wrist. The tactile surface of the palm may function similarly to the extended receptor surface (retina) of the eye, with wrists muscles corresponding to eye muscles (MacKenzie & Marteniuk, 1985). Realignment should develop in the same manner as for the eye–head system if the coordination task affords stimulation of the extended tactile receptor surface. ·

We make the simplifying assumption that when an intrasystem misalignment occurs the anomalous system is unlinked from other systems until the misalignment can be removed by concerted action in the anomalous system. However, the consequence of intrasystem realignment is to produce an intersystem misalignment. The local noetic space of the anomalous system will be out of register with the noetic space of other systems. Intersystem misalignment is removed when misaligned systems are coordinatively linked to perform a common task.

Intersystem Misalignment

An experimental example of intersystem discordance is the case in which a wedge prism is mounted in front of the eye via goggles and subjects are required to engage in eye–hand coordination tasks (e.g., Redding & Wallace, 1988b; Uhlarik & Canon, 1971). The eye can successfully foveate any target in the visual field, and there is no intrasystem discordance. However, noetic coordinates of a target encoded by the eye–head system will conflict with the noetic coordinates required for the hand to achieve the target; that is, intersystem discordance (see Fig. 4.3). Removal of intersystem discordance involves the same kind of cooperative realignment of both exteroceptor and proprioceptor encoders described for intrasystem discordance, only now the adapting system is under external rather than internal control.

Initially, the hand may move to the position indicated by the eye–head system but will miss the target because of the error in visual encoding induced by the prism. Note carefully that missing the target per se does not produce discordance or realignment. The hand achieves the commanded position more or less accurately and there is no local discrepancy in the hand–head system with the expected position (corollary discharge). In the usual experimental case, where there is no input from an extended tactile receptor surface such as the palm of the hand, the collateral (Fig. 6.1) picks out the noetic coordinates expected for tactile input, but there is no discordance detection and realignment in the exteroceptor encoder.

Discordance detection and realignment in the proprioceptor encoder arises when attempts at correcting the error are made based on visual feedback—the observed difference between hand and target positions. Reissuing a position command would produce the same error, but a difference command can reduce the error. The local hand–head system feedback controller transfers the prescribed difference code to the hand (effector) via the decoder, but the expected position (corollary discharge) to the proprioceptor encoder remains expressed as a position code. When the hand achieves the commanded position, that position conflicts with the expected position. This discordance motivates a gradual realignment in the proprioceptor encoder of the hand to agreement with signal from the remote eye–head visual system. Thus, misalignment is between target noetic coordinates expressed by the remote guiding system and noetic coordinates required by the local guided system to achieve the target. But discordance detection and realignment occurs locally in the guided system.

In the case just described, the entire load of aligning the hand–head with the eye–head system would be carried by the proprioceptor encoder in the hand–head system. Adaptive change in the exteroceptor encoder requires an extended receptor surface such that target position in exteroceptor space can be experienced simultaneously with effector position in proprioceptor space. The normally small tactile field makes realignment in touch unlikely. Such exteroceptor realignment is more likely to occur for visual and auditory systems with larger sensory fields, especially when corrective movement of the effector via difference commands (feedback control) is prevented.

If extended tactile input is available, the kind of cooperative realignment of both exteroceptor and proprioceptor function described for intrasystem discordance will occur. Consider the case where the subject's task is to center the palm of the hand over a visually given target and the subject can feel the raised target against the palm. The hand will initially achieve the visually given position with no discrepancy between encoded hand position (proprioceptor output) and expected hand position (corollary discharge). But the collateral will disagree with the tactually encoded target position (exteroceptor output) with consequent realignment in the tactile sense. If corrective movements of the limb are not made, realignment will be restricted to the exteroceptor encoder. With corrective movements, realignment will also occur in the proprioceptor encoder.[7]

In the examples just discussed, the direction of coordinative linkage is eye-to-hand; the hand responds to and is guided by the eye. Consequently, discordance is detected locally in the hand–head system and realignment is restricted to this system (Generalization 4, chapter 4). The outcome will be different if the coordination task requires the reversed direction of linkage, in which target position is first specified by the hand–head system and used to guide the eye–head system (e.g., in the everyday task of looking at one's wristwatch). Now, discordance detection and realignment will be localized in the eye–head system, with the same kind of cooperative realignment of encoders outlined for the guided hand–head system. The normally extended nature of visual (retinal) input in the eye–head system enhances the likelihood of localized realignment in the exteroceptor encoder, but the substantially reflexive nature of corrective eye movements assures that the larger part of realignment will usually be localized in the proprioceptor encoder.

These examples of intersystem discordance detection result in realignment of eye–head and hand–head systems, but, of course, misalignment with other spatial systems (e.g., ear–head). Such distortions of noetic space can only be maintained for any extended period of time in artificial exposure environments that constrain changes in the direction of coordinative linkage. The frequent shifts in the direction of guidance linkages among the various sensorimotor systems required by everyday tasks assures ultimate convergence on cross-alignment of the entire perceptual–motor system.

Depending on the directional linkages required by everyday coordination tasks, realignment will reverberate among the various components of the perceptual–motor system until the entire system settles into a veridical state of cross-alignment. At any point in time, the total state of alignment for the system will be the simple algebraic sum of local realignment in subsystems (Generalization 4, chapter 4). Of course, the magnitude of each kind of local realignment will also depend on the unique dynamic characteristics of each adaptive encoder, but estimation of these parameters is an empirical problem.

---

[7]These predictions have not been tested. Investigations of tactile input on adaptation to prismatic displacement has produced disappointingly small effects (e.g., Welch, 1978). However, these studies did not provide stimulation of an extended tactile surface like the palm of the hand. Neither did they test for change in tactile position maps, for example, by having the subject verbally indicate when a tactile stimulus is centered on the palm of the hand.

SUMMARY

Spatial alignment of sensorimotor representations is mediated by a common noetic representation. General transformational operators map positions in sensory (exteroceptor) space and motor (proprioceptor) space onto corresponding positions in noetic space. The inverse mapping of noetically coded commands onto motor space enables effector action. For spatially aligned systems, the task-specific exchange of calibration signals among the hierarchically organized sensorimotor elements establishes the present condition of the task–work space in noetic terms. Such calibration permits movement planning and evaluation.

When spatially misaligned sensorimotor elements are coordinated under feedback control, these calibration signals do not pick out corresponding positions in noetic space. The resultant discordance stimulates a long response time, incremental change in transformation parameters to realign sensorimotor representations with noetic space and, therefore, with each other. Such realignment will be localized in the guided system established by higher level planning functions. Depending on response to error feedback, realignment may be localized for sensory or motor space. Only online feedback control with error information from an extended-field exteroceptor can establish the necessary conditions for misalignment detection and consequent realignment.

Chapter 7

THEORETICAL ISSUES

Two primary theoretical questions in prism adaptation are concerned with the nature of adaptation (what changes?) and the conditions under which adaptation occurs (when does the change occur?). In this chapter, we discuss these issues in the context of the theoretical framework developed in chapters 5 and 6. This chapter also provides a more detailed justification of the context (chapter 4) for the present model.

First, we suggest how a third adaptive process, postural adjustment, may be distinguished from strategic control (chapter 5) and spatial realignment (chapter 6). In our discussion of the nature of adaptation, we further address the longstanding question of whether visual realignment is a change in retinal local sign or in eye position sense. This question is related to the more general provision in chapter 6 for exteroceptor and proprioceptor realignment and some empirical predictions are developed. We then discuss the traditional issue of whether prism aftereffects have their origin in changes in or between eye and hand systems. We show how adaptive change between these sensorimotor system can be identified with strategic control and motor learning, whereas realignment is identified with adaptive change in sensorimotor systems. We conclude the first section of the chapter with a summary illustration of how postural adjustment, strategic control, and spatial realignment are related in eye–hand coordination.

Second, we discuss how conditions known to be conducive of prism aftereffects can be understood in the present theoretical framework. Previous research and theory regarding the importance of active movement is interpreted as facilitating direct coordinative linkage of misaligned sensorimotor systems and, therefore, enabling misalignment detection and consequent realignment. The role of exposure performance error is then considered in terms of how various error-correction strategies can affect misalignment detection and reduction. Finally, in this section we discuss the effects of selective attention in terms involving controlled processes to retrieve task-specific coordination strategies that determine the locus of realignment. We also show how coordination strategies may fail to link misaligned sensorimotor systems under conditions of high cognitive load.

We conclude this treatment of theoretical issues with a discussion of possible sources of limitation on the realignment process. We distinguish between structural limits imposed by the evolutionary history of the organism and process limits imposed by the combined operation of multiple adaptive mechanisms. Conditions are identified under which postural adjustment and strategic control can limit realignment. In particular, we show how the conditions that give rise to intersensory dominance (especially, visual capture) may preclude misalignment detection and consequent realignment.

THE NATURE OF ADAPTATION

How is a person different after adaptation to prisms? What has changed to enable adaptive behavior? There is surely no single answer to this question. Adaptive behavior is a composite of spatial realignment, strategic control (skill learning), and postural adjustment. To defend the thesis that spatial realignment is a uniquely important part of the total adaptive response, it must be shown to be theoretically and methodological distinct. Thus, the goal in this section is not to deny other contributions to adaptive behavior but rather to show how spatial realignment stands in relation to other adaptive changes as a unique and essential part of the total adaptive response.

We begin by contrasting postural adjustment with spatial realignment. We then examine the traditional question of whether visual realignment has it basis in exteroceptor (retinal local sign) or proprioceptor (eye position sense) functions. Next, we discuss the issue of adaptive change between sensorimotor systems (strategic control) versus adaptive change in sensorimotor systems (realignment). We conclude this section by showing how the three kinds of adaptive change are related in the eye–hand system.

Postural Adjustment

Simply adopting an atypical body posture during prism exposure can enable adaptive behavior. For instance, turning the head in the direction of lateral optical displacement serves to center the optical flow pattern in the visual field and facilitates locomotion (Redding & Wallace, 1988c). Of course, discordance between head position in motor space and head position indicated by the centered optical flow could serve as the basis for a realignment of the head position sense, but a change in the head position sense could also arise simply from the atypical posture. The apparently simple nature of postural adjustment belies its processing complexity. Ebenholtz (1974, 1976; Ebenholtz & Fisher, 1982; Paap & Ebenholtz, 1976, 1977) articulated a mechanism for such adaptive postural change that attributes prism aftereffects to more peripheral processes in motor space.

Ebenholtz (1974) began with the observation that after a prolonged period of isometrically or isotonically asymmetric exertion against an external load such as gravity or an obstacle to movement, apparently relaxed muscle continues to be innervated. This continuing innervation causes an involuntary movement in the direction normally associated with the previous exertion. For example, after leaning against a wall, supporting one's self by pressing the back of the wrist against the wall, or after simply holding the arm extended against the pull of gravity for a period of a minute or two, the relaxed arm will involuntarily move outward and up away from the body. It is as if a running average of patterned innervation is fed back and added to momentary innervation, producing residual muscle potentiation.

Such residual innervation is assumed to be "reflexive in the sense that it cannot be compensated for and is the mechanical equivalent of a hidden load attached to the muscles" (Ebenholtz, 1974, p. 477). Thus, the set-point or resting position of the effector is shifted in the direction opposite the load with no corresponding change in position signaled by the proprioceptor. Normally, such a mechanism might serve to compensate for directional loading without the necessity for changes in central programming. For instance, prolonged exposure to a constant gravity field may induce compensatory muscle potentiation, enabling the limb to achieve a constant position in response to the same centrally issued command whether the movement is made with or against gravity.

This muscle-potentiation mechanism is possibly implicated whenever a muscle system receives exercise that is asymmetric about the body midline; that is, even when there is no external load. Successful coordination of sensorimotor systems in any prism exposure situation necessitates that at least one motor system be asymmetrically exercised. Consequently, muscle potentiation may produce adaptive changes in effector position with predictable position sense aftereffects.

According to this postural adjustment hypothesis, intersystem misalignment is not a cause of prism adaptation but is only one way of establishing the necessary conditions for muscle potentiation. Ebenholtz and coworkers (1976; Ebenholtz & Fisher, 1982; Ebenholtz & Wolfson, 1975) demonstrated the expected postural aftereffects in oculomotor and neck muscles (see also Craske, Crawshaw, & Heron, 1975; Howard & Anstis, 1974), and the same mechanism may be responsible for prism aftereffects in other sensorimotor systems (see Craske, 1981).

However, prism aftereffects have also been demonstrated under conditions of arguably symmetrical exercise (Craske & Crawshaw, 1974, 1978) and even in the direction opposite that predicted by asymmetrical posture (Redding & Wallace, 1988c). Thus, it would seem that both postural adjustment and spatial realignment are adaptive mechanisms that contribute to the total adaptive response. Figure 7.1 illustrates how the two mechanisms might be related in the present theoretical framework.

Figure 7.1(A) illustrates a possible postural adjustment mechanism. The efferent command is a position code in motor (M) space expressed as a pattern of agonist–antagonist activation necessary to achieve the desired position. For instance, the simplest kind of pattern might be the difference between agonist innervation (I_a) and antagonist innervation (I_t). Efference ($I_a - I_t$) is compared with the set point or reference value to determine the change in relative magnitude of agonist–antagonist innervation needed to place the effector in the desired position. Sign operators on the output of the comparison reflect reciprocal inhibition of the muscle pair.

The relative magnitude of actual agonist–antagonist innervation is assumed to be fed back and integrated over time (Σ) to determine the momentary set point value.

(A)

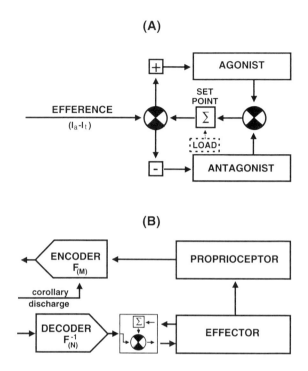

(B)

FIG. 7.1.   Adaptive postural adjustment. (A) Patterned innervation is averaged and added to momentary innervation. Such muscle potentiation is compensatory in the sense that following a prolonged period of exertion against a load, a constant position can be achieved in response to the same centrally issued command whether the movement is made with or against the load. Even in the absence of load, as in prism exposure, asymmetric exercise produces residual asymmetric innervation. This hidden load results in adaptive changes in effector position with predictable perceptual aftereffects. (B) This load compensator is shown positioned in motor space on the efference side of a sensorimotor system in relation to adaptive encoding–decoding operators (see also Fig. 6.1).

When an effector is loaded, the relative magnitude of agonist–antagonist innervation is adjusted by feedback to achieve or maintain the commanded position. Conversely, temporal integration assures that the correspondence between actual and commanded positions will be reachieved following load removal.

Prism exposure activates this load compensator by imposing a period of asymmetric exercise that alters patterned innervation with corresponding shifts in actual effector position for commanded positions. Return to symmetric exercise will restore correspondence between actual and commanded position.

Postural aftereffects of prism exposure, therefore, reflect the adaptive capacity of the motor system to adjust to changing load, but this capacity does not obviate the need to detect environmental change (e.g., load) and to realign the encoding function that maps motor onto noetic space. Indeed, such load compensation produces misalignment with other components of the perceptual–motor system and, in the case of a temporally extended load, creates a need to realign encoding functions.

Figure 7.1(B) illustrates how the load compensator (simplified by collapsing over agonist–antagonist innervation) may be positioned relative to the adaptive alignment mechanism (compare with Fig. 6.1). Thus, postural adjustment is a more immediate solution to the problems created by changing load whereas realignment is the more long-term solution. Such adaptive changes in posture can be methodologically distinguished from adaptive alignment in a particular sensorimotor system by establishing conditions of symmetrical exercise of that subsystem (Craske & Crawshaw, 1974, 1978; Redding & Wallace, 1988c).

Exteroceptor and Proprioceptor Realignment

A longstanding issue in prism adaptation is whether realignment occurs in sensors that code position in extrapersonal space (exteroceptors) or is restricted to position sensors in intrapersonal space (proprioceptors). An early form of this question was whether realignment is localized in proprioceptive systems such as the hand–arm or in the visual system (Harris, 1963, 1965; Rock, 1966). The development of modality-specific tests (e.g., Hay & Pick, 1966b) demonstrated that adaptive alignment can be visual or proprioceptive in nature depending on certain conditions (e.g., Rock & Harris, 1967).

However, the fact that the appearance of the visual world changes does not directly address the question of exteroceptor versus proprioceptor realignment. Such phenomenal change in vision might arise from either change in the head-centric significance of retinal loci (exteroceptor realignment) or change in eye-position sense (proprioceptor realignment). Consequently, the present focus is on the nature of realignment in sensorimotor systems, especially the visual system.

The few studies that have directly addressed the question of retinal local-sign change in adaptation to prismatic displacement (Cohen, 1966; Crawshaw & Craske, 1974; Howard, 1971a) have produced equivocal results (for a review see Welch, 1978). Several studies support oculomotor shift, showing change in felt direction of gaze following exposure to prismatic displacement (Craske, 1967; Kalil & Freedman, 1966; McLaughlin & Webster, 1967; Webster, 1969), but this result is also subject to alternative interpretation (see Kornheiser, 1976; Lackner, 1973; Rock, 1966).

Change in felt direction of gaze could itself arise from changes in retinal local-sign or in felt head position (see Welch, 1978, for a summary of these arguments). Moreover, head-centric visual realignment to transformations like optical rotation (Ebenholtz, 1966; Redding, 1978) is not readily explicable in terms of eye-position sense realignment because the eye may not be capable of torsional movements of sufficient magnitude.[1] Mikaelian (1990) argued against a postural adjustment explanation for such tilt realignment. Thus, whether visual change involves exteroceptor or proprioceptor realignment is an open question.

---

[1]For reviews see Howard (1982) and Howard and Templeton (1966).

The uncertain state of evidence bearing on the question of exteroceptor versus proprioceptor realignment arises from the lack of theory sufficiently developed to enable contrasting predictions. The present theoretical framework provides the basis for such tests by making provision for both kinds of realignment.[2] More specifically, manipulation of the error-corrective response should affect the relative magnitude of exteroceptor and proprioceptor realignment in the eye–head system.

To illustrate, assume a situation in which the direction of guidance linkage is hand-to-eye, wherein the unseen hand is specified as the target for a visual locational response (Howard, Craske, & Templeton, reported in Howard & Templeton, 1966). The subject looks to where his hand feels to be and, when visual position of the hand is made available, the subject should register discordance, and realignment should occur in the eye–head system, but this adaptation may be a change in the head-centric significance of retinal loci or in the eye-position sense depending on whether a corrective movement of the eye is made.

To see why this is so, assume that Fig. 6.1 represents the eye–head system under remote guidance by the hand–head system; that is, the eye is positioned to correspond to the position of the unseen hand. Now, consider what happens when the hand is viewed through displacing prisms; that is, when visual feedback is provided, but the two systems are optically misaligned.

Prior to any corrective eye movement and assuming continued hand-to-eye guidance linkage, there should be discordance between the encoded afference and the calibration signal in the exteroceptor (retina) encoder but not in the proprioceptor (extraocular muscles) encoder. The corollary discharge originating in the hand–head system specifies, say, a straight ahead position for the hand and the eye will be in that position within precision limits, having achieved it prior to viewing the optically displaced hand. Thus, there should be no discordance and adaptive change in the proprioceptor (extraocular muscles) encoder. However, the hand will not be foveated but will be seen displaced (i.e., via the retinal exteroceptor afference). Thus, the collateral of the eye position sense will signal straight ahead while the encoded retinal signal will specify a displaced hand position with resultant discordance and realignment of exteroceptor (retina) encoder.

On the other hand, the motivation for adaptation will be reversed for the two visual system encoders after a corrective eye movement has been made to zero-out the error; that is, after a relative-position (difference code) command based on the retinal difference between fovea and seen hand positions. The corollary discharge continues to signal a straight-ahead hand position as demanded by its calibration role, but the encoded extraocular afference (i.e., proprioceptor input) signals a displaced hand position, with resultant discordance and realignment in the proprioceptor encoder. Meanwhile, the displaced hand position signaled by the collateral of encoded proprioceptor afference (i.e., extraocular muscles) agrees with the encoded retinal signal, thereby removing the motivation (discordance) for realignment of exteroceptor (retinal) encoder.

---

[2]See also the discussion of intrasystem discordance in chapter 6.

In the usual situation in which corrective movements are permitted, even required, adaptation may be largely or entirely a change in the proprioceptor spatial mapping function. It is not surprising, therefore, that changes in effector position are usually associated with adaptation (Craske, 1967; Kalil & Freedman, 1966; McLaughlin & Webster, 1967; Webster, 1969). However, manipulations that delay or even prevent corrective responses may enhance exteroceptor realignment and overt changes in effector position may not accompany such adaptation. These two kinds of realignment may also be parametrically distinguishable, because exteroceptor and proprioceptor encoding functions may be expected to have different temporal characteristics. For such parametric comparisons, however, the same directional guidance linkage must be maintained to avoid confounding intrasystem with intersystem realignment.

The present theoretical framework provides a basis for distinguishing between exteroceptor versus proprioceptor realignment. Our focus is on the traditional instance of this question in the visual system, but the question need not be so restricted. Similar predictions might be made concerning the consequences of corrective hand movements for realignment of exteroceptor function (tactile position sense) and proprioceptor function (limb position sense) when the hand–head is the guided system, provided spatially extended stimulation of tactile receptors is available.

Coordination

Postural adjustment and exteroceptor or proprioceptor realignment in sensorimotor systems are parts of the total adaptive response to misalignment among parts of the perceptual–motor system. Adaptive changes may also occur between sensorimotor systems, in those processes that produce common action of the various parts of the total perceptual–motor system. Two related proposals characterize such adaptive coordination as sensorimotor adaptation (Efstathiou, Bauer, Greene, & Held, 1967; Hardt et al., 1971) and adaptive change in coordinators (Templeton et al., 1974; Welch, 1974).

Work from Held's laboratory (Efstathiou et al., 1967; Greene, 1967; Hardt et al., 1971) suggests that adaptation can occur for coordination of sensorimotor systems without accompanying adaptive changes in the component systems. For example, Hardt et al. (Experiment 2) found a significant eye–hand coordination aftereffect following prism exposure but no evidence of change in the hand or eye position senses. Change in the hand position sense was measured by having subjects place their unseen hand in remembered positions learned prior to prism exposure. Change in the eye position sense was measured by intermanual transfer of altered target pointing from the exposed to the unexposed hand. Remembered-position results have proven difficult to replicate (Craske & Gregg, 1966; Kennedy, 1969; but see Efstathiou et al., 1967), and the validity of intermanual transfer as a measure of visual realignment is questionable (Redding & Wallace, 1988b). Nevertheless, such results raise the possibility that coordination processes can account for part of the total adaptive response of the perceptual–motor system to misalignment.

In the present model, adaptive coordination (strategic control) takes the form of planned intervention by higher level processes that monitor coordinative linkage of sensorimotor systems (chapter 5). The planner (Figs. 5.1 and 6.1) is assumed to have available a variety of strategies, including the ability to override normally direct coordinative linkage between systems and to exercise more deliberate control. Movement plans can deliberately specify positions for the guided system that do not match target positions indicated by the guiding system. In this manner, adaptive behavior can be achieved over successive trials during prism exposure even though realignment is incomplete.

For example, in eye–hand coordination, a person may point not where a target looks to be, but at a position to the side of the target where the finger will be on target when it comes into view. With practice, such a side-pointing strategy may become sufficiently established to transfer to similar coordination tasks following exposure. In effect, the guided system is placed in remembered positions learned during exposure and not in positions directly given by the guiding system. This strategy means that misaligned systems are effectively unlinked and discordance registration and reduction (i.e., realignment) will not occur.[3]

To the extent that such deliberate control is exercised, it may appear on aftereffect tests without evidence of local realignment in component sensorimotor systems. Such an unlinking strategy would be particularly encouraged by the extensive pretraining of remembered positions employed by the Held group.

Adaptive strategies in coordination correspond to what has been variously called *adaptation at complex sites* (Welch, 1978) or *adaptive change in coordinators* (Howard, 1971b; Templeton et al., 1974). The contrast here is with adaptation at simple sites or realignment. An important prediction from such a hierarchical view of perceptual–motor organization is that "changes in lower coding elements necessarily affect tasks involving elements higher in the system, but changes in higher elements do not affect tasks involving only lower elements" (Templeton et al., 1974, p. 249; see also Wilkinson, 1971).

If adaptation occurs at both simple and complex sites, the total adaptive change measured for a perceptual–motor system like the eye–hand system should exceed the sum of adaptive changes measured separately for component sensorimotor systems like the eye–head (visual) subsystem and the hand–head (proprioceptive) subsystem. Such underadditivity (Redding & Wallace, 1978) is observed under conditions that may be expected to encourage the kind of adaptive coordination strategy suggested by the present model—namely, target pointing where error feedback is available (Redding & Wallace, 1988b; Templeton et al., 1974; Welch et al., 1974). Moreover, Templeton et al. found that underadditivity decreased when error feedback is terminated, consistent with the present view that adaptive coordination (strategic control) and realignment are fundamentally different processes.

The source of underadditivity in these studies was characterized as motor learning (Welch, 1978; Welch et al., 1974), but this seems an incomplete descrip-

---

[3]See also the discussion of Knowledge of Results Compensation in chapter 5.

tion. To learn an adaptive motor response during prism exposure, the person must discriminate a visual position that would correct for the observed pointing error and then strategically intervene in direct coordinative linkage to send this position, *not* the target position, to the hand. Strategy implementation, as well as motor learning, seem to be involved. Welch's motor learning seems to be the same kind of process as Held's sensorimotor adaptation.

The present model provides for adaptive coordination (strategic control), as distinct from either postural adjustment or spatial realignment, and identifies position training and error feedback as conditions that encourage this kind of adaptation. Like postural adjustment, adaptive coordination is a more immediate solution to the performance problems posed by misalignment, whereas realignment is the long-term solution. In the prism adaptation paradigm, contributions of adaptive coordination can be detected by the additivity test. Adaptive coordination is estimated by the difference between total adaptive change and the sum of adaptive change in component subsystems of a perceptual–motor coordination loop.

Eye–Hand System

Figure 7.2 summarizes, for the eye–hand system, the three mechanisms for adaptive change proposed by the present model. For many coordination tasks, the eye–hand system is assumed to be analyzable into two functional sensorimotor subsystems, spatially referenced on the head: eye–head and hand–head subsystems.

In each subsystem, load compensators for eye and limb–neck muscles (effectors) produce adaptive postural adjustments in response to externally imposed load or prolonged asymmetrical exercise (Fig. 7.1). Also in each subsystem, encoders that translate between sensorimotor (S–M) spaces and mediating noetic (N) space, respond adaptively to discordance between input and calibration signals (corollary discharge and collateral) with gradual realignment to remove spatial misalignment between subsystems (Fig. 6.3). Strategic coordination (control) is illustrated by optional connections through the planner.

Common action of eye and hand is usually realized by direct coordinative linkage, in which spatial coordinates of targets are exchanged. With such direct linkage, spatial misalignment detection and realignment will occur in the guided subsystem. The linkage direction shown in Fig. 7.2 would produce localized realignment in the hand–head system. However, in unusual situations, such as large spatial misalignment of eye and hand, successful performance may require mediated linkage, in which the spatial coordinates passed between subsystems are those needed to minimize performance error, not those of corresponding spatial positions. With such mediated linkage, realignment will not occur, although the eye–hand system will show adaptive behavior.

Note that load compensators are activated solely by asymmetric exercise of effectors. Asymmetric exercise may be elicited by spatial misalignment or chosen in the course of action planning, but neither adaptive alignment or strategic coordination mechanisms directly affect such postural adjustment.

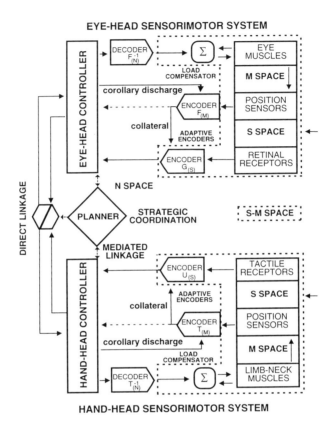

EYE-HEAD SENSORIMOTOR SYSTEM

HAND-HEAD SENSORIMOTOR SYSTEM

FIG. 7.2. The eye–hand system. In each component sensorimotor system are illustrated adaptive postural adjustment on efference (Load Compensators) and adaptive realignment of Exteroceptor and Proprioceptor afference (Encoders). Adaptive coordination (strategic control) processes are illustrated by the optional connections of the planner, especially direct connections to subsystem controllers.

Figure 7.2 illustrates the assumed relationship among three theoretically distinct components of adaptive perceptual–motor coordination: adaptive alignment, strategic coordination, and postural adjustment. We have shown how this framework can suggest methodological as well as theoretical distinctions. We now turn to consideration of the conditions under which these kinds of adaptive change can occur, especially adaptive alignment.

CONDITIONS FOR REALIGNMENT

Different kinds of adaptation require different conditions. The conditions for adaptive coordination involve all the complexities of motor control and learning (see chapter 5). In contrast, the necessary and sufficient conditions for postural adjustment and spatial realignment are relatively simple. Postural adjustment occurs whenever a sensorimotor system is asymmetrically exercised, and factors that affect the duration and extent of asymmetrical positioning will affect postural adjustment. Spatial realignment is the automatic response to discordant spatial information, and all conditions that promote realignment in one way or another enable discordance detection (chapter 6). In this section, we indicate how known conditions for realignment (active movement, performance error, and selective attention) may be related in the present theoretical framework.

Reafference

Clearly, the minimal condition for realignment is that the person be provided with information in some form about the nature the misalignment of systems. The most influential and successful hypothesis about the conditions for realignment is the idea that the requisite information must be derived from active bodily movement (Held, 1961; Held & Hein, 1958). Figure 7.3 illustrates Held's model of the visuomotor system in a manner that facilitates comparison in the present theoretical framework.

According to this model, when a motor act such as eye or hand movement is initiated, an efferent copy of the command is held in correlational storage and becomes associated via an afferent collateral with the visual consequence of the movement (reafference). The development of this efferent–reafferent trace enables the current efference to retrieve expected reafference that can then be compared

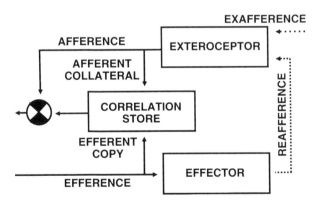

FIG. 7.3.   The reafference hypothesis. *Reafference* (produced by self-movement) is distinguished from *exafference* (produced by object movement) by comparison of expected movement selected from memory (Correlation Store) by the Efferent Copy with actual movement (Afference). Under normal conditions, the Comparator output is zero producing a stable perceptual world with self-movement. Under distortion conditions, new correlations between efference copy and corollary discharge are laid down, reducing Comparator output and restoring a stable perceptual world. Adapted from "A Neural Model for Labile Sensorimotor Coordinations" by A. Hein and R. Held. In E. E. Bernard and M. R. Kane (Eds.), *Biological Prototypes and Synthetic Systems* (p. 74), 1962, New York: Plenum. Copyright 1962 by Plenum. Adapted with permission.

with current reafference to determine further performance. A mismatch would normally indicate objective position change in the visual field (an exafferent signal), calling for appropriate compensatory motor behavior.

For example, active exploratory movements of the eye or hand (reafference) in response to movement of objects (exafference) would elicit a difference signal from the comparator, reflecting change in object position and indicating appropriate response. With active bodily movement in the absence of exafference, expected and current reafference would match and the zero output of the comparator would signal a stable visual world. With change in the world (exafference) in the absence of a reafferent signal (passive movement or a static effector), there would be no output from the correlation storage to cancel exafference and the comparator would signal objective position change. With neither reafference or exafference, comparator output would be zero. The model thereby enables detection of changes in visual stimulation arising from movement of objects in the world by canceling out stimulation arising from self-movement. Note that the lack of a consistent relationship between efference and exafference assures that spurious correlation will not develop.

Now, when a distorting device is placed in front of the eyes, the normal efference–reafference correlation is no longer present. Movement of the hand or eyes retrieves expected reafference that does not match the current visual reafference and the afferent signal is interpreted as exafference. Phenomenally, the limb may appear to be moved by some external force, or the entire visual world may appear to move when the eyes move. If there is a consistent relationship between efference and reafference, however, a gradual recorrelation of efferent outputs with the new reafferent inputs occurs and the system recovers its ability to distinguish exafference from reafference. In the meantime, while the recorrelation is being established, the output of the comparator is used to modify motor behavior (e.g., eye or limb movements) as if the signaled difference indicates exafferent events (e.g., world movement or external load). Such comparator output prior to recorrelation accounts for response error early in prism exposure.

As a model of perceptual–motor coordination, Held's proposal differs in several substantive ways from the present one. Perhaps the most global difference is in the scope of the two proposals. Held's model is restricted to accounting for visuomotor coordination wherein the visual exteroceptor guides various effector systems such as extraocular and limb muscles and makes no provision for other directions of linkage among other sensorimotor systems. The model also provides only for realignment of the visual exteroceptor and is not directly capable of accounting for proprioceptor realignment (e.g., the eye position sense) or realignment in other sensorimotor systems (e.g., the limb position sense).

Perhaps because of this limited scope, communication among sensory and motor spaces in Held's model is mediated by visual space. The correlation store can be viewed as a device for expressing positions in motor space in the coordinates of visual space. Retrieval of associated reafference amounts to an expression of the motor command represented by the efferent copy in visual coordinates. In this way, sensory and motor positions can be compared in common coordinates to determine appropriate behavior.

Not shown in Held's model, but necessary for its operation, is an inverse device to change visual into motor coordinates on the efferent side. Thus, any extension of the model would have to face the problem of the limited representational capacity of visual space. Moreover, the associative nature of the translation between spaces means that the assumed relationship between sensory and motor space is an arbitrary one. The transformational operators of the present proposal embody the more likely assumption (Bedford, 1989) that relationships among the several spaces of the perceptual–motor system are constrained by physical geometry (chapter 3).

Furthermore, Held's model is solely a mechanism for coordinating response with changes in object position (perceptual–motor coordination) and does not provide for any representation of the perceptual world (MacKay, 1973). The subtractive role of the efferent copy means that the comparator only detects exafference and outputs no signal in the absence of changes in the world. No information is provided that could form the basis for a perceptual map of the world (Rock, 1966). Without such a perceptual representation, behavior would be a succession of responses to successive object movements, a neverending chase, with no possibility of purposeful, goal-directed behavior like reaching for or foveating a stationary object.

In contrast, the present proposal provides for parallel transfer of information from all locations on a receptor surface, forming a representation of the receptor's field. The assumed interpretive role for calibration signals (chapter 6) assures that sensory information is properly categorized as to source (exafference or reafference) without any loss of information and is expressed in coordinates usable by higher level coordinative and perceptual processes.

Finally, an empirical limitation of Held's model is the strong prediction (reaference hypothesis) that active bodily movement is a necessary condition for adaptation.[4] With passive movement or a stationary effector, there is no efferent copy to associate with the afferent collateral and no recorrelation can occur.[5]

The reafference hypothesis was initially supported by a variety of studies that showed that prism aftereffects occurred with active movement but not with passive movement (Held & Bossom, 1961; Held & Freedman, 1963; Held & Gottlieb, 1958; Held & Schlank, 1959). However, subsequent studies by other investigators generally failed to replicate the absence of aftereffects with passive movement, although passive movement may produce smaller aftereffects (Baily, 1972; Fishkin, 1969; Foley & Maynes, 1969; Pick & Hay, 1965; Singer & Day, 1966; Weinstein, Sersen, & Weinstein, 1964). Moreover, active movement does not ensure that aftereffects will occur (Wallace & Garrett, 1973, 1975). Thus, active movement is neither a necessary nor sufficient condition for realignment (Welch, 1978).

In our proposal, at least one kind of realignment can occur with stationary effectors. Realignment is the automatic response to persistent discordance between

---

[4]Weaker predictions are possible (Held & Mikaelian, 1964), but the reafference hypothesis remains the strongest test of the model.

[5]Indeed, the absence of output from correlation storage would assure that the comparator would always interpret passive changes in body part position as arising from objective changes in the world, a dissociation of sensory and motor functions

continuously available afferent and calibration information. Calibration signals must be continuously available because of their interpretative role in determining present position.[6] Exteroceptor afference is also continuously available. Thus, at least in the form of exteroceptor realignment, adaptation can occur even with stationary effectors. Data from some previous studies are consistent with this interpretation (Howard, Craske, & Templeton, 1965; Kravitz & Wallach, 1966).

Also in this proposal, active movement is not sufficient for realignment. The necessary condition for intersystem realignment is that sensorimotor systems be coordinatively linked so that discordance information is available to drive realignment of adaptive encoders, but this linkage need not be active in the sense of intentional effector movement. Direct coordinative linkage and consequential realignment is more likely with active movement. But sensorimotor systems can function autonomously without being coordinatively linked or systems may be linked indirectly, mediated by higher level strategic considerations. In either case, active movement occurs without intersystem misalignment detection and realignment.

Performance Error

Another condition that is conducive of prism aftereffects is the presence of explicit targets during exposure. The total shift[7] aftereffect in eye–hand coordination is greater with visual targets, even with passive limb movement (Baily, 1972; Freedman, 1968; Melamed, Haley, & Gildow, 1973; Templeton, Howard, & Lowman, 1966).

This target-pointing effect (Welch, 1978), however, is not solely a matter of more salient discordance afforded by an explicit landmark. Total shift is greater when subjects experience and subsequently correct target-pointing errors compared to target-pointing without error (Coren, 1966; Welch, 1969, 1971b; Welch & Abel, 1970; Welch & Rhoades, 1969). Even error-correction may not be necessary. Significant total shift occurs when the correct response is practiced without experiencing a significant error (Dewar, 1971; Howard et al., 1974; Jakobson & Goodale, 1989; Templeton et al., 1974; Uhlarik, 1973). The target-pointing effect, therefore, arises from the opportunity to practice the correct response afforded by explicit target.

There is evidence, however, that the presence of explicit targets induces a motor learning component in the total shift. With explicit exposure targets, total shift in eye–hand coordination tends to be greater than the sum of adaptive changes in the eye–head and hand–head systems (Beckett, 1980; Beckett, Melamed, & Halay, 1975; Redding & Wallace, 1978; Templeton et al., 1974; Welch et al., 1974).

---

[6]See the previous discussion of calibration in chapter 6.

[7]This aftereffect is assessed by target pointing without sight of the pointing limb and was originally called the *negative aftereffect*. We prefer *total shift* because it is now clear that such negative aftereffects usually reflect the sum of aftereffects that have their source in component eye–head and hand–head systems.

Moreover, the presence of explicit targets affects the magnitude of total shift without affecting adaptive shift in eye–head or hand–head subsystems (Redding & Wallace, 1988b).

Therefore, practicing the correct response enhances a motor learning component of adaptation without being necessary for realignment. Such motor learning may be the sole basis for the target-pointing effect. However, we argued in chapter 6 for a more complex relationship between performance error and realignment: Error-free performance produces maximal realignment of motor space, but uncorrected performance error produces the conditions for realignment of sensory space. We now discuss this relationship between performance error and discordance.

Performance error and spatial discordance are distinct kinds of information, serving different needs of the perceptual–motor system. Performance error serves controllers (Fig. 5.3), enabling corrective movements to acquire a target and learning of the correct response. Discordance serves adaptive encoders (Fig. 6.3), enabling detection of misalignment and realignment of spatial mapping functions. The two kinds of information operate at different levels. However, because encoders are hierarchically subordinate to controllers, performance error and discordance can have interactive effects. Variables that affect coordinative linkage may also affect realignment because spatially misaligned sensorimotor systems must be coordinatively linked for discordance detection and realignment to occur. In particular, performance error and correction can indirectly affect realignment by determining the manner in which misaligned systems are coordinatively linked.

Some of the complexity of the interaction between strategic control and adaptive alignment is suggested by how the perceptual–motor systems may identify error sources. Error in intersystem coordination can arise either from encoding of target position by the guiding system or from execution of the response by the guided system. Errors of either type normally arise from inherent imprecision or from environmental changes such as target movement or change in effector load. In any case, the source of the error must be determined before corrective measures can be undertaken. Such error identification involves strategic reversal of the directional linkage between systems, initiated by higher-level planning functions.

For example, in eye-to-hand coordination (visual guidance), when the limb fails to achieve the position of the visual target, identification of the error can be achieved by reversing the linkage between systems. Hand-to-eye proprioceptive guidance provides the eye–head controller (Fig. 5.3) with information about limb position that can then be compared with its previously issued position command. If a match is found, then the error arose from faulty encoding of target position. Eye-to-hand linkage is then reestablished, the eye–head controller reencodes target position, perhaps with a corrective foveating eye movement for greater precision, and reissues a new position command to the hand–head system.

On the other hand, if a mismatch occurs, then the error arose from faulty execution on the part of the hand–head system. Eye-to-hand linkage is reestablished and a corrective command is issued to the hand–head system in the form of a difference coded command to zero-out the error. Such error identification and correction and practice of the correct response normally serves to refine sensory and motor parameters in skill learning and would enhance this component of the total adaptive response to prismatic distortion.

A similar source-of-error analysis using only visual information (i.e., exclusive visual guidance) could be applied if the only source of error was normal imprecision. In this case, the called-for correction is a repeat of encoding or execution with increased precision. Greater precision, however, would not enable correction of errors arising from slowly developing, normally small, spatial misalignments among subsystems. Spatial alignment errors may require more deliberate correction strategies such as perhaps slightly pointing to the side of where the target looks to be, and execution of such strategies requires information about limb position. To acquire this information requires hand-to-eye linkage. Because misalignments are natural events, it seems likely that error identification processing normally involves bidirectional exchange of information between eye–head and hand–head subsystems.

Even for ostensibly visually guided eye-to-hand coordination tasks, error-identification processing assures some reversed hand-to-eye coordinative linkage. Consequently, some local realignment will occur in both eye–head and hand–head systems under conditions of prismatically induced misalignment.

Position information from the hand–head system may be used as the calibration signal in the eye–head system. Subsequent comparisons both motivate eye–head realignment and provide information that the hand has deviated from the intended position. (Phenomenally, the limb appears to have been influenced by some external environmental force). Such information is used as the basis for a difference coded command to make in-flight corrections or corrections in limb position after the primary movement has been completed. In this case, the position command to the hand–head system remains unchanged, providing for continued discordance detection and realignment in the hand–head system. Alternatively, the information may be used to unlink the systems and deliberately point to the side of the target on the next movement. When the systems are deliberately unlinked, however, the motive for hand–head realignment is removed.

Under conditions that discourage error correction the normally short duration, hand-to-eye, error-identification linkage may be prolonged to dominate coordination of eye–head and hand–head systems. For example, when sight of the limb is delayed until the primary movement is completed and secondary corrective movements are prohibited, limb position information may be used to guide the following eye, and realignment will be predominantly localized in the eye–head system. Alternatively, if errors are saliently large, as when an explicit visual target is present, a deliberate side-pointing strategy may be employed. The systems will be unlinked and the strategic control contribution will be large (i.e., the target-pointing effect), but realignment will be reduced.

Note carefully that neither error identification or error correction is an obligatory process, although the latter presupposes the former. A person may choose not to attend to error information if it is available or not to act on such information. Still, position information from one subsystem can be used to automatically initiate movements by another subsystem. Such automatic coordinative linkage establishes the conditions for realignment.

For some coordination tasks, error identification routines may not be well developed and may, therefore, require extensive monitoring by higher level planning functions. In such cases, error identification may not occur if higher level processes are otherwise occupied. Error correction does not occur unless the source of error is identified. Nevertheless, exteroceptor realignment can occur even without error correction so long as the misaligned systems are coordinatively linked.[8]

Given that error identification occurs, error correction still may not occur. Whether the corrective movement is made depends on higher level decision processes that evaluate the acceptability of the error in the error tolerance requirements of the present task (Proteau, 1992). Small errors may well be tolerated as good enough for the task at hand. Under such conditions, some realignment of both exteroceptor and proprioceptor functions will occur in the guided system.

Selective Attention

Several studies have implicated selective attention in realignment. Canon (1970, 1971) proposed that when two spatial modalities provide discrepant information about a distal object, it is the unattended modality that is realigned. For example, Canon (1970) directed attention to one modality by instructing the subject to track with the right hand either the prismatically displaced visual target or the pseudo-phonically displaced auditory target during exposure. The conflict between visual and auditory location was resolved by realignment of the unattended modality.

Kelso et al. (1975) found that if attention is directed to the proprioceptive modality by specifying the left hand as the target for a right hand pointing response during prism exposure, realignment was entirely restricted to the visual modality. But when attention was directed to visual targets only proprioceptive realignment of the left hand–head system occurred.

Similarly, Uhlarik and Canon (1971) argued that visual eye–head realignment is greater when sight of the pointing limb is delayed until the end of the pointing movement because the subject's attention is mainly directed toward the proprioceptive information from the arm during its unseen excursion. In contrast, proprioceptive hand–head realignment is greater when both visual and proprioceptive information are concurrently available over the entire course of the pointing movement because attention is concentrated on the available visual input.

These observations can be summarized by saying that realignment tends to occur in the unattended modality. In this context, however, the term *attention* is purely descriptive rather than explanatory, and the essential idea is better expressed in terms of the exposure task's particular demand structure that determines the guided and guiding subsets of the total set of sensorimotor subsystems (Redding, 1979; Redding et al., 1985).

This is most clearly true of Canon's theoretical position. Perception is assumed to be based on efferent signals evoked by association with afferent stimulation

---

[8]This assumes that the exteroceptor function is not experimentally amputated, for example, by preventing sight of the limb or tactile input.

(Festinger et al., 1967; Taylor, 1962). Realignment occurs in the guided system (unattended modality), because the afference from this source is discrepant with the efference originating in the guiding system (attended modality). There is no such efference–afference discrepancy for the guiding modality and thus no adaptation.

The Kelso, Cook, Olson, and Epstein (1975) theoretical position can also be interpreted in similar terms. Perception is assumed to be based on the consensual significance of simultaneous afferent sources (see also Epstein & Morgan-Paap, 1974). In the case of conflict between afferent sources, resolution is achieved by realignment of the guided system (subordinate source) to agree with the guiding system (situationally dominant source). The structure of the exposure task, including instructions, therefore, determines the guiding modality whose function *must* remain unchanged for successful task performance (Hamilton, 1964; Howard & Templeton, 1966, p. 380).

These effects of task structure are realized in the present proposal by changes in the direction of coordinative linkage between sensorimotor systems. Explicit instructions as well as implicit task structure such as feedback availability determine how subsystems are coordinated to perform a task. When spatially misaligned systems are coordinatively linked, the spatial discordance between systems is detected in the guided system, which is then realigned to agree with the spatial coordinates of the guiding system.

For example, if subjects are instructed to point at a visual target (visual guidance instructions), the coordinative linkage is eye-to-hand and discordance registration and realignment occurs in the hand–head proprioceptive system. Conversely, if subjects are instructed to look at their hand (proprioceptive guidance instructions), the linkage is hand-to-eye and realignment occurs in the eye–head visual system.

If visual feedback is delayed until the end of a pointing movement, subjects are forced to rely on available proprioceptive feedback (hand-to-eye proprioceptive guidance) and realignment is largely visual in nature. But, if visual and proprioceptive feedback are concurrently available over the course of the pointing movement, subjects use the available visual information (eye-to-hand visual guidance) and realignment should occur predominantly in the proprioceptive system.

To the extent that task structure permits or requires changes in the direction of coordinative linkage between misaligned systems, realignment should occur in all systems implicated in the task.[9] The use of the term *attention* to describe these effects only creates an illusion of explanation. It does not add any explanatory or predictive power beyond that which can be better achieved by a careful delineation of the task structure specifying the direction of guidance (Redding, 1979; Redding et al., 1985). The present model, however, incorporates a more substantive meaning for attention (see also chapter 1).

The direction and timing of coordinative linkage is strategically determined in response to characteristics of the coordination task. A variety of plans are available for dealing with different situations. Strategies differ in the amount of effort

---

[9]See also Generalization 4 in chapter 4.

required for execution (Hasher & Zacks, 1979; Kahneman, 1973; Posner & Snyder, 1975; Schneider et al., 1984; Schneider & Shiffrin, 1977a).

Some habitual coordination plans can be executed with little conscious effort, requiring little more than a simple intention to make a movement. Such automatic linkages are relatively fast and make few demands on the limited capacity of the planner to monitor their execution. Other less common tasks require more deliberate effort to control their execution. Such controlled linkages are relatively slow and place greater demands on limited central processing capacity. For instance, proprioceptive guidance (hand-to-eye linkage) may be an uncommon, more controlled process requiring slow movements, whereas visual guidance (eye-to-hand linkage) may be a routine, more automatic process and occurring with faster movements. Also, automatic processes tend to be mandatory whereas controlled processes are more optional.

Depending on the level of analysis, automatic versus controlled processing is not a dichotomous distinction (Shiffrin & Dumais, 1981). At a molecular level of analysis, parts of a process may be controlled whereas other parts are automatic (Schneider & Fisk, 1983). For instance, eye–hand coordination tasks may involve a synchronized mixture of largely automatic visual guidance and more controlled proprioceptive guidance. Moreover, even in largely automatic visual guidance, error analysis and correction may involve more controlled processes.

Thus, coordination of sensorimotor systems is constrained to the extent that monitoring a particular linkage draws on limited central processing capacity or attention.[10] Because coordinative linkage of misaligned systems is necessary for discordance detection, realignment may not occur if monitoring capacity is not available. In particular, realignment that depends on controlled linkage of misaligned systems is subject to interference from secondary cognitive tasks that preempt central processing capacity.

For example, in eye–hand coordination tasks, realignment of the visual system that depends on more controlled proprioceptive guidance is subject to cognitive interference. Realignment of the proprioceptive hand–head system that depends on more automatic visual guidance is less affected by a secondary cognitive load. And, to the extent that error correction is a controlled process, exteroceptor realignment may occur under cognitive load.

LIMITS ON REALIGNMENT

A hundred years of research with the prism adaptation paradigm reveals amazing plasticity in the perceptual–motor system. The same research has also suggested limits on the adaptive process. In the present theoretical framework, we can distinguish between structural limits that are imposed by the evolutionary history of the organism and process limits that are imposed by the combined operation of multiple adaptive mechanisms.

---

[10]For reviews, see Klein (1976) and Stelmach (1982). See also chapter 1.

Structural Limits

Perceptual processing is likely constrained by the nature of the physical stimulus (Marr, 1982; Shepard, 1984), and structural limits on realignment may reflect these physical constraints. For instance, Bedford (1989; especially Experiment 4) found evidence of a linear constraint on realignment of visual eye–head and proprioceptive hand–head subsystems. Following exposure to curvilinear misalignment of visual and proprioceptive spaces, adaptive aftereffects reflected a linear solution for the misalignment, with change in both slope and intercept. It is important to note that in Bedford's procedure exposure to misalignment is restricted to at most three corresponding visual–proprioceptive locations, but the resulting realignment tended to extend across the entire visual–proprioceptive map, including untrained locations (see also Bedford, 1993a, 1993b).

The observed linear constraint reflects the kind of general transformational operators assumed for adaptive encoders (chapter 6; see also chapter 3). Only a few studies have explored the nature of such constraints on spatial mapping operations (Cunningham, 1989; Hay, 1974; Hay, Langdon, & Pick, 1971) and methods for isolating particular encoding operators for study have only just begun to be developed (Bedford, 1989; Redding, 1973a, 1975b).

Another possible source of structural limits is the response rate of the adaptive encoder. For instance, Ebenholtz and Callan (1980; see also, Ebenholtz & Mayer, 1968) estimated for tilt realignment that maximal gain (proportional adaptation) is attained for an input rate (increasing tilt) of about 1.4 deg/min. Increasing tilt at faster rates produced proportionally less realignment. Thus, high input rate may overdrive the system, exceeding the structurally given response rate of the adaptive encoder and interfering with realignment. Different encoders may have different response rates that reflect the rate at which misalignment naturally occurs.

Process Limits

When people first experience an optical transformation such as tilt or displacement of their visual field, they show obvious behavioral difficulty. For instance, in reaching for objects, they miss the intended target, and they tend to be hesitant and to stumble when walking. However, usually in a few minutes, these obvious errors disappear. The person appears to have adapted to the distorted visual stimulation. Perceptual–motor behavior during exposure appears to be adaptive even though aftereffect measures of realignment may show incomplete compensation for the distortion (Redding & Wallace, 1993). With few exceptions (Baily, 1972; Hay & Pick, 1966a), the maximum obtained realignment does not even approach complete compensation for the distortion (Ebenholtz, 1966; Efstathiou, 1969; Hay & Pick, 1966b; Redding, 1973b). Complete realignment is usually found for only a few selected subjects (Hein, 1972; Held & Bossom, 1961; Mikaelian & Held, 1964).

In the majority of cases, realignment seems to become asymptotic and short of being complete, no matter how long the exposure period. For instance, with optical tilt up to about 30 deg, realignment appears to be asymptotically limited at about

25% of the distortion in the first 5 min. of exposure (Ebenholtz & Callan, 1980). Such limits on realignment do not appear to be structural in nature because realignment does occur and is asymptotically limited even for small distortion magnitudes at low input rates. Rather, such limitations appear to be inherent in the adaptive process itself.

In our theoretical framework, process limits on realignment are explained by other components of the total adaptive response (postural adjustment and strategic control), that, at the same time, support adaptive behavior and reduce detected discordance. For instance, a change in effector set-point will enable achievement of the position signaled by a remote guiding system without local discordance detection. Detected discordance and resultant realignment are reduced by postural adjustment. Also, depending on whether a corrective movement is made in a guided sensorimotor system, discordance registration will occur in proprioceptor or exteroceptor. Realignment of the other encoding function is therefore limited.

Strategic unlinking of misaligned systems will also enable adaptive behavior but reduce discordance detection and produce apparent limits on realignment. The proportional decrease in realignment for large distortions (Dewar, 1970; Ebenholtz, 1973; Ebenholtz & Callan, 1980; Ebenholtz & Redding, 1970; Efstathiou, 1969; Miller & Festinger, 1977) may occur because extreme distortion makes input unrecognizable as a basis for guidance of another system. Under such conditions, the misaligned systems may not be coordinatively linked and realignment will be reduced (Ebenholtz & Callan, 1980; Rock, 1966). Adaptive behavior may also be mediated by indirect linkage of aligned systems, such as when a side-pointing strategy is employed. Without activation of the direct linkages necessary for discordance detection, realignment will be reduced (Redding, 1981; Redding & Wallace, 1993).

Another example of limits on realignment imposed by strategic control is illustrated by intersensory bias (dominance) effects. The immediate effect of viewing the hand through displacing prisms is that the hand comes to feel where it looks to be. When vision and proprioception are in conflict, vision tends to dominate, to capture proprioception. Welch (1978, 1994; Welch & Warren, 1980; Welch et al., 1979) argued that such visual capture of felt limb position is antithetical to realignment.[11] Figure 7.4 illustrates this position in our theoretical framework.

When two sensorimotor systems can be assumed to signal the same spatial position, spatial information from either system could be used to guide a third sensorimotor system. For example, when only the left limb is visible, right-handed pointing at the left hand could be guided by either the seen or felt left hand position. Choice of guiding system is strategically dependent on ecological reliability. For example, visual position is usually more reliable and may be chosen more frequently than proprioceptive position. The eye–head system may be coordinatively linked with the right hand–head system.

Phenomenal experience is dependent on coordinative linkage. Unused position information is not generally passed to higher centers that mediate phenomenal

---

[11]For a contrasting view, see Epstein (1975), Epstein and Morgan (1970), and Wallach (1968).

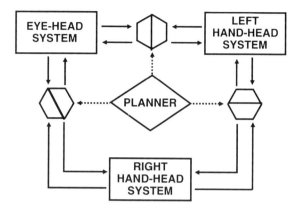

FIG. 7.4. Intersensory Bias (especially Visual Capture). When the stationary left hand is viewed through distorting prisms, the ecologically more reliable visual position dominates phenomenal experience and is used to guide a pointing response with the unseen right hand. To the degree that such visual capture occurs, the eye–head and left hand–head systems are unlinked, and discordance detection and realignment are reduced.

experience. Therefore, the phenomenal consequence of preparing a right-hand response is that the left hand is experienced where it looks to be. When visual and proprioceptive systems are misaligned by displacing prisms, the result of such coordinative linkage is visual capture. The right hand pointing will be guided more by seen than felt left-hand position.

Note carefully that eye–head and left hand–head systems are not linked, discordance between these systems cannot be detected, and there is no basis for realignment. Moreover, the measurement of intersensory bias effects (see Welch & Warren, 1980) requires that the responding right-hand system not be visible. Discordance between eye–head and right hand–head systems cannot be detected, and there is again no basis for realignment.

The strategic control processes involved in selecting from among several sources of spatial information may effectively unlink misaligned systems and produce limited discordance detection and realignment. Of course, subjects may exercise directional guidance between discordant systems and show realignment aftereffects, but this represents a failure of procedure to constrain behavior to the intersensory bias paradigm.

One way in which this might happen is if the subject is required to actively position the effector in one or both of the conflicting systems. Active movement encourages directional guidance. To the extent that active movement of conflicting systems is required, guidance signals may be exchanged between these systems and realignment may occur.

On the other hand, passive positioning of the hand may encourage less direct guidance linkage between the conflicting systems and the response system, especially because the visual information is not available from the response system.

Thus, passive movement tends to produce large intersensory bias effects, whereas active movement tends to produce large realignment effects (Welch et al., 1979).

Welch and Warren (1980) identified a variety of factors that affect the magnitude of intersensory bias and that may reflect planner action in the present model. The action of the planner governs which of the two conflicting systems is in momentary control of the third response system. Rapid switching of coordinative linkage between the two conflicting systems results in an intermittent mix of signals that are integrated by the response system controller. This averaged signal is biased in the direction of the most frequently sampled of the two conflicting systems.

To the extent that planner operation involves controlled processing, a secondary cognitive task imposed simultaneously with the primary task should reduce intersensory bias effects. However, limited processing capacity is only one factor affecting planner operation and exact predictions about the effects of cognitive load requires taking into account the ecologically based strategies available to the planner.

The intersensory bias paradigm seems ideally suited to determining the parameters of planner operation. Because such characteristics of the planning function contribute to determining the direction of coordinative linkage between systems, it should be possible to predict the relative magnitude of local realignment from a knowledge of intersensory bias effects.

SUMMARY

Three kinds of adaptive processes have been distinguished: realignment of the spatial mapping onto noetic space of sensory space (exteroceptor) or motor space (proprioceptor), postural adjustment in the resting level of innervation (set-point) to agonist-antagonist muscles, and strategic control to enable common action (coordination) of sensorimotor systems.

Because detection of discordance requires direct coordinative linkage of misaligned sensorimotor systems, the locus and magnitude of realignment depends on factors (active movement, performance error, and attention) that determine task-specific coordination strategies.

Realignment is limited not only by structural features such as the valid spatial transformations and response characteristics of adaptive encoders, but also by the contributions of other adaptive processes (postural adjustment and strategic control) to the total response of the organism.

PART III

RESEARCH

We now turn to empirical tests of the view of prism adaptation developed in the preceding four chapters. In chapters 8 and 9 we summarize our research that has been guided by the theoretical framework developed in chapters 5 and 6. In chapter 10 we develop some implications for future research and theory. In these chapters, we stress the distinctions among the three kinds of adaptive perceptual–motor processes: spatial alignment, strategic control, and postural adjustment.

Most prism-adaptation research has employed various eye–hand coordination tasks (for reviews, see Welch, 1978, 1986). Such coordination readily lends itself to a variety of controlled manipulations, and in chapter 9 (Adaptive Eye–Hand Coordination) we describe some studies that employ this procedure to perform an experimental analysis of the components of adaptive spatial behavior, especially realignment. However, the analytical power of eye–hand coordination procedures also entails the largely unknown risk of producing laboratory situations that are so artificially restricted that they have limited generalizability to more natural situations.

Another experimental tradition in prism-adaptation research is less susceptible to this criticism (Ebenholtz, 1966; Kohler, 1951/1964). Free locomotion during exposure to optical distortion of visual input is arguably less artificial and provides empirical evidence of ecological validity for theories of adaptive spatial alignment. Moreover, because it is more difficult to control experimentally such exposure tasks, greater articulation of theory is necessary to identify relevant variables. One of our goals has been to explain adaptive behavior under locomotion conditions. Our manipulations have been limited by the need to preserve the natural integrity of the exposure situation. In chapter 8, Adaptation During Locomotion, we review these attempts to understand adaptive spatial alignment during locomotion.

Chapter 10, Implications, concludes this monograph first by summarizing the most important theoretical distinctions suggested by our analysis of prism adaptation: multiple adaptive processes, basic sensorimotor systems, and different kinds of learning. We show how the prism adaptation paradigm can address these theoretical issues and make specific suggestions for further research. We conclude with a brief summary of our theoretical framework for adaptive perceptual–motor performance.

Chapter 8

ADAPTATION
DURING LOCOMOTION

Our initial development and test of the present model employed the paradigm of relatively unrestricted locomotion about natural human environments (hallway exploration). In this research, we focused on the role of coordinative linkage of sensorimotor systems in producing realignment during locomotion. First, we tested the hypothesis that coordinative linkage of the misaligned visual system with other sensorimotor systems requires intentional effort. When attention is distracted by a secondary cognitive task, coordinative linkage will not be established with the consequence that discordance detection and realignment aftereffects will be reduced. Then, we tested among the several possible directional linkages to determine which one(s) were critical for realignment. Finally, controls were introduced to exclude adaptive changes in eye and head posture as the sole basis for prism aftereffects. Throughout this research, we have checked for additivity of realignment components to provide a measure of contributions from strategic control.

METHODOLOGY

In all of these studies, subjects walked about common institutional hallways for short periods of time with the distorting optical device mounted in front of their eyes. The exposure period was typically 10 minutes, and the distortion was usually prismatic displacement. The only restraint on behavior was that subjects were instructed not to engage in orienting or manipulatory eye–hand behavior with objects in the environment.

Aftereffect measures were obtained to focus on spatial realignment in the eye–head visual system and the hand–head proprioceptive system. For the visual shift (VS) test, subjects were instructed to adjust (usually by verbal instructions to the experimenter) a visual target to appear straight ahead of the nose without error feedback or knowledge of results. For the proprioceptive shift (PS) test, subjects were instructed to point straight ahead of the nose without sight of the hand or knowledge of results.

Because the VS and PS tests are referenced to the head, comparisons of performance on these tests before and after prism exposure provide measures of adaptive change in the eye–head and hand–head systems, respectively. Moreover, because these aftereffect tests are performed without error feedback or knowledge of results and are very dissimilar to locomotion behavior required during exposure, they are arguably measures of realignment rather than strategic control (see also chapters 4 and 7).

A total shift (TS) aftereffect measure was obtained by having subjects point at a visual target without sight of their limb or knowledge of results before and after prism exposure. Including this test enables assessment of additivity; VS + PS = TS. Because the TS test is sensitive to any adaptive change in systems inclusive of eye and hand, deviation from additivity can be taken as an indicator of adaptive strategies deployed during prism exposure that transfer to the aftereffect tests.

COGNITIVE LOAD

We first tested the cognitive interference prediction (Redding et al., 1985; Redding & Wallace, 1985a). In the prism exposure situation, normally automatic linkages between spatially misaligned sensorimotor systems produce performance errors. Reestablishment of accurate behavior requires deliberate strategic control. Accurate performance in the prism exposure situation requires allocation of limited central processing capacity to establish and maintain error-corrective linkage between systems. It follows that if central processing capacity is not available, discordant systems will not be linked, exposure performance will suffer, and realignment aftereffects will not appear. This prediction has been tested in a number of experiments employing the hallway exposure procedure.

The general strategy was to compare aftereffects for differently treated groups of subjects. All subjects were required to walk about hallways viewing a world laterally displaced 17.1 deg. In addition, experimental subjects were also required to simultaneously perform a secondary cognitive task like mental arithmetic with hallway exploration. The usual aftereffect tests of visual and proprioceptive realignment and total shift were administered before and after a 10 min hallway exposure.

Figure 8.1 shows the results of one of these experiments (Redding & Wallace, 1985a). There were four groups of 15 subjects each. A control group did not receive a secondary task. Three experimental groups received mental-addition problems of increasing difficulty: single-digit problems, double-digit problems with double-digit answers, and double-digit problems with triple-digit answers. As can be seen, both visual aftereffects (VS) and proprioceptive aftereffects (PS) decreased steadily as the percentage of correct problems decreased. As expected, realignment suffered from cognitive interference. The more difficult the secondary task, the more central processing capacity was required and the less capacity was available to link discordant systems. Consequently, realignment decreased in a graded fashion with increasing secondary task difficulty.

This result was replicated many times, for both optical rotation (tilt) and displacement, and under a variety of conditions to exclude alternative explanations (Redding

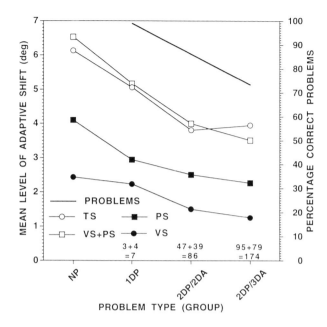

FIG. 8.1. Cognitive interference in prism adaptation. Level of visual shift (VS) and proprioceptive shift (PS) and percentage of correctly solved mental addition problems (PC) as a function of four levels of problem difficulty: no problems (NP), single-digit problems (1DP), double-digit problems with double-digit answers (2DP-2DA), and double-digit problems with triple-digit answers (2DP-3DA). Examples of problem types are shown at appropriate points along the abscissa. Also shown are Total Shift (TS) for comparison with the sum of visual and proprioceptive components (VS + PS). From "Cognitive Interference in Prism Adaptation," by G. M. Redding and B. Wallace, 1985a, *Perception and Psychophysics, 37*, p. 227. Copyright 1985 by Psychonomic Society, Inc. Adapted with permission.

et al., 1985). For example, interference with realignment is not greater when the secondary task involves a larger mental imagery component. It does not seem to be the case that realignment is reduced because the secondary task preempts perceptual mechanisms (Farah, 1989; Segal & Fusella, 1970), thereby reducing information pickup. Moreover, as illustrated in Fig. 8.1, the total adaptive change in the eye–head system (TS) was not different from the sum of visual aftereffects (VS) and proprioceptive aftereffects (PS). Aftereffects are completely accounted for by realignment in component eye–head and hand–head systems.

COORDINATIVE LINKAGE

What are the coordinative linkages evoked during locomotion that suffer interference from cognitive load, with consequential reduction in realignment? In this section, we report our explorations of possible linkages of the visual system with locomotive foot–head, proprioceptive hand–head, and auditory ear–head systems.

Locomotive and Visual Systems

The visual realignment shown in Fig. 8.1 might have arisen from discordance between spatial positions indicated by the locomotive foot–head and visual eye–head sensorimotor systems. Visual feedback in the form of optical flow produced by movement along the hallway might signal a spatial position different from that indicated by eye position. For example, if the direction of movement signaled by center of the optical expansion pattern is taken to indicate egocentric straight-ahead, then this position indicator will be displaced from the straight-ahead position indicated by center of the visual field. If information derived from locomotion is used to guide locational movements of the eye, the local discordance detected in the eye–head system would prompt realignment of visual coordinates with consequential aftereffects. And if such foot-to-eye linkage requires intentional control, then secondary cognitive load would reduce the frequency of linkage and, therefore, the amount of visual realignment.

This foot-to-eye linkage hypothesis was evaluated by comparing level of realignment aftereffects for different walking rates. If optical flow is involved in realignment, then the more salient optical flow produced by faster walking rates should increase the amount of realignment. In a variety of conditions, however, walking rate has been shown to be unrelated to realignment (Redding et al., 1985; Redding & Wallace, 1985a, 1985b).

For example, in one experiment subjects walked as fast as possible, back and forth down the center of a short hallway while wearing displacing prisms (Redding & Wallace, 1985b, Experiment 1). They were instructed to fixate a large target at each end of the hallway, walk rapidly toward it, and to close their eyes while making an about-face turn at each end. Walking rate was high at about 63 m/min. Many subjects had to be constrained from running down the hallway. Optical flow was surely exaggerated. Nevertheless, realignment of the eye–head (or hand–head) system did not occur. Locomotion per se and associated optical flow do not seem to be involved in realignment. Cognitive interference with realignment cannot be explained by reduced optical flow information arising from lower walking rates under cognitive load.

Moreover, the high walking rate that can be attained suggests that visual guidance of locomotion (i.e., eye-to-foot coordinative linkage) is not affected by optical displacement of the visual field. The precise effect of optical displacement on optical flow is problematic because the nature of the information extracted from optical flow is not completely understood (Cutting, 1986; Larish & Flach, 1990; Longuet-Higgins & Prazdny, 1980). However, it is easy to see how motion information might be insulated from optical displacement.

The pattern of optical flow need not be centered in the visual field in order to be a useful indicator of direction of self-movement. Indeed, under normal conditions, head movements frequently produce peripherally positioned flow patterns with no noticeably detrimental effect on locomotion. And, under optical displacement, optical flow can easily be centered in the visual field by adopting an asymmetric head posture, not unlike what normally occurs. Also, rate of self-movement and obstacle proximity indicators in optical flow are unlikely to be affected by largely uniform transformations of the visual field like optical displacement and rotation.

Finally, visual guidance of locomotion seems to be an automatic process, not substantially affected by cognitive load. The natural tendency for subjects to walk more slowly while performing mental arithmetic is easily countered by instructions. For instance, for the data displayed in Fig. 8.1, subjects in all of the experimental groups received instructions that encouraged and *produced* faster walking (averaging 52.7 m/min) than the control group (38.4 m/min). Thus, subjects can easily be encouraged to use the available visual information to support rapid locomotion even under cognitive load (Redding et al., 1985; Redding & Wallace, 1985b). Note also that this observation provides further evidence against the idea that visual realignment arises from foot-to-eye coordinative linkage. The experimental subjects walked faster, experiencing more salient optical flow, and still showed reduced realignment.

In summary, walking rate has not been found to be related to either realignment or performance of the secondary cognitive task in a variety of conditions. These results suggest that control of locomotion is automatic and based on information derived from self-movement, which is unaffected by such optical transforms as lateral displacement and rotation of the visual field. Walking rate does not suffer interference from cognitive load because the relevant visual information is not distorted and locomotion can be guided in the usual automatic manner. Walking rate does not affect realignment because the optical flow derived from self-movement does not provide positional information that can be discordant with the positional information distorted by the optical transform. The positional significance of retinal stimulation is transformed by optical displacement, but information about self-movement provided by optical flow is not distorted. Locomotion is guided by distinct motion-sensitive channels that are not affected by the optical transformation.[1]

Proprioceptive and Visual Systems

The realignment of proprioceptive hand–head and visual eye–head systems shown in Fig. 8.1 may have been produced by strategic changes in the direction of coordinative linkage between proprioceptive and visual systems that are encouraged by structural aspects of the exposure situation. For example, the hallway wall on the side in the direction of the optical displacement appears to be farther away than it actually is. Subjects frequently bump the wall with their shoulder. These proprioceptive encounters can provide discordance information that may prompt realignment of the hand–head system, even though subjects obeyed instructions not to actively touch the wall with their hand. Subjects first see the looming wall, anticipate an encounter with their shoulder, and when the encounter occurs sooner than expected, the feedback is an occasion for detecting the discordance

---

[1]Aftereffects of rearranged optical flow on location (Rieser, Pick, Ashmead, & Garing, 1995) may reflect associate transfer of calibration among functionally similar perceptual–motor systems rather than arise from realignment.

between "seen" and felt positions of the shoulder.[2] The direction of coordinative linkage is eye-to-hand, subjects feel for the wall with their shoulder, and the discordance detection and realignment occurs in the hand–head system (proprioceptive shift).

The reverse direction of coordinative linkage could be responsible for visual realignment if subjects are not attending to the visual position of the wall. If they do not register where the wall is in anticipation of a proprioceptive encounter, then bumping the wall may be an occasion of visual search for the obstacle based on proprioceptive information. Subjects look for the wall where their shoulder tells them it is located. The direction of coordinative linkage is hand-to-eye and discordance between felt and seen location of the wall provides a basis for realignment in the eye–head system (visual shift).

Support for this interpretation of the sources of realignment during hallway locomotion comes from a study in which displacement direction was factorially combined with near-wall position (Redding & Wallace, 1988c). Different groups were instructed to walk near the left wall or near the right wall while wearing prisms that displaced the visual field in either the leftward or rightward directions. Proprioceptive realignment appeared in the right hand–head system only when conditions afforded frequently anticipated proprioceptive encounters; that is, when subjects were instructed to walk near the right wall with rightward displacement. Visual realignment of the eye–head system, however, tended to appear in all conditions, even when proprioceptive encounters with the wall were infrequent. When subjects were instructed to walk near the right wall with leftward displacement, the wall appeared closer than it actually was but subjects usually avoided collisions. Therefore, we looked elsewhere for a more substantial basis for visual realignment.

Auditory and Visual Systems

A clue to another source of visual realignment was provided by the unexpected finding shown in Fig. 8.1 that proprioceptive aftereffects were greater than visual aftereffects. Visual realignment is usually greater than proprioceptive realignment in hallway exposure conditions (Redding et al., 1985). However, these previous experiments were conducted in hallways with noisy human traffic. The data in Fig. 8.1 were collected from some of the same hallways, but the occupants of offices in that area had been serendipitously evacuated in preparation for renovation. Consequently, the frequency of subject encounters with visible sound sources was much reduced. We hypothesized that this might account for the reversal in relative magnitude of the two kinds of realignment.

Auditory encounters could produce visual realignment in the following manner: Subjects first hear a sound source and then direct their eyes and head to look at the

---

[2]Note carefully that the discordance is not between phenomenal seen and felt positions. Phenomenal experience is assumed to arise from a higher level of processing. Neither is discordance between visual and proprioceptive systems. Misalignment occurs between systems, but as shown in chapter 6, detection of misalignment (discordance) is the function of low-level encoders in the guided system which compare expected position (calibration signal) with achieved position (encoded afference). "Seen," "felt," or "heard" position is only a convenient shorthand for describing this more primitive process in sensorimotor systems. For further discussion, see Redding and Wallace (1995b).

sounding target. The direction of coordinative linkage between auditory ear–head and visual eye–head systems would be ear-to-eye. Heard position is used to guide the searching eye. The discordance between auditory and visual positions would be registered in the visual system, prompting realignment of the encoding operators in the eye–head visual system.

This ear-to-eye linkage hypothesis was tested by manipulating the availability of visible sound sources. In one experiment, the only systematically available sound source was the speaking experimenter, setting mental arithmetic problems for the subject (Redding & Wallace, 1985b, Experiment 3). In different conditions, the experimenter either walked behind the subject and was not visible, or stood at the end of the hallway and was visible to the subject as the problems were given. Also, the mental arithmetic problems were either easy (single-digit) or difficult (double-digit). Thus, the design provided for assessment of the independence of factors involving task structure (visibility of sound sources) and cognitive load (problem difficulty). Cognitive load should affect the subjects' ability to coordinatively link sensorimotor systems and, therefore, the overall level of realignment. Task structure should affect the direction of coordinative linkage between misaligned systems and, therefore, the locus of realignment.

The principle results of this experiment are displayed in Fig. 8.2. As can be seen, the larger cognitive load produced by double-digit problems was equally effective in producing less of both kinds of realignment. Realignment was largely

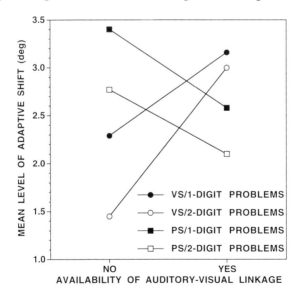

FIG. 8.2. Auditory-to-visual coordinative linkage. Level of visual shift (VS) and proprioceptive shift (PS) as a function of the availability of coordinative linkage between visual and auditory systems. When the speaking experimenter could not be seen by the subject, no auditory–visual linkage was available, but when the experimenter was visible, such linkage was possible. Data are also shown for different groups receiving single-digit and double-digit problems (data are from Redding & Wallace, 1985b).

visual in nature when the visible experimenter made the auditory–visual linkage available. These results confirm the independence of cognitive load and task structure factors and the importance of auditory-to-visual linkage in producing visual realignment.

In the absence of visible sound sources, subjects activate predominantly eye-to-hand coordinative linkage, anticipating proprioceptive encounters with the visible wall, with consequential large proprioceptive realignment. But, when visible sound sources are available, subjects attempt to look at them, activating ear-to-eye linkage, producing largely visual realignment. Finally, it should be noted that TS and VS + PS had identical values in all conditions, indicating that these tests were sensitive to realignment without contamination from control strategies deployed during exposure.

POSTURAL ADJUSTMENT

Postural adjustment is an alternative to realignment as an explanation of after-effects following hallway exposure (Ebenholtz, 1976; see also previous discussion in chapter 7). For instance, if the eyes are asymmetrically positioned during exposure, then visual shift aftereffects might be due entirely to change in the resting position for the oculomotor muscles. Similarly, if the head is asymmetrically positioned during exposure, then proprioceptive shift aftereffects might be entirely due to change in set point for the neck muscles. The contribution of postural adjustment to adaptation during locomotion has been assessed by manipulating conditions that can be assumed to affect the degree of asymmetric eye and head posture (Redding & Wallace, 1987, 1988c). The basis for prediction is illustrated in Fig. 8.3.

If the head is kept straight during hallway exposure, the eyes must turn in the displacement direction to look in the direction of locomotion; that is, to fixate the center of the expansion pattern. Such asymmetric eye posture could cause a shift in resting eye position such that in the visual aftereffect test, a visual position actually displaced in the direction of the previous optical displacement would be judged straight ahead of the nose. Thus, eye posture aftereffects would appear on the visual aftereffect test.

If the head is kept straight, the visual appearance of the hallway is much as it would be if the head were turned in the base direction, opposite the direction of displacement. There would be discordance between visual information about head position and felt head position that would form the basis for realignment of the head–neck system. Such realignment of head position would cause subjects, in the proprioceptive aftereffect test, to feel their straight head to be turned in the base direction. To point straight ahead of the nose, subjects would point in the direction opposite the displacement. Therefore, with the head straight, there is a basis for both postural aftereffects in the eye–head system and realignment aftereffects in the head–neck system.

However, if the head is turned in the displacement direction, the eyes will tend to be straight in the head, reducing the basis for postural aftereffects in the eye–head system, but creating a basis for postural aftereffects in the head–neck system. Thus,

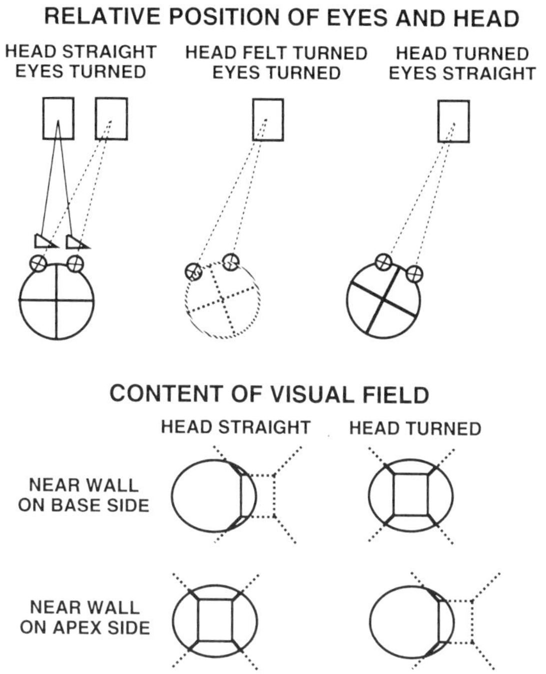

RELATIVE POSITION OF EYES AND HEAD

HEAD STRAIGHT   HEAD FELT TURNED   HEAD TURNED
EYES TURNED   EYES TURNED   EYES STRAIGHT

CONTENT OF VISUAL FIELD

HEAD STRAIGHT   HEAD TURNED

NEAR WALL
ON BASE SIDE

NEAR WALL
ON APEX SIDE

FIG. 8.3. Body positions during hallway exposure. Optical displacement (prism base left, rightward displacement) of the hallway may induce a felt head rotation (prism base direction) with the eyes turned (displacement direction) in the head or an actual head rotation (displacement direction) with the eyes straight in the head. The visual image of the hallway will be centered in the visual field only when the head is turned (displacement direction) and the subject stands near the wall on the base side or when the head is straight and the subject stands on the apex (displacement) side of the hallway.

depending on whether the head is straight or turned in the displacement direction during prism exposure, postural aftereffects are possible in the eye–head or hand–head systems, respectively.

In fact, the head is not usually kept perfectly straight during locomotion with displacing prisms. There is a tendency to turn the head in the displacement direction (Kohler, 1951/1964). Such head turning is largest when subjects are near the wall on the base side of the prisms (opposite the displacement direction) because all they may see without turning their head is the near wall (see Fig. 8.3). Head turning is less when subjects walk near the wall on the displacement side (apex of the prism) because the structured visual array and direction of locomotion tends to be centered in the available visual field (that is restricted by the prism bearing goggles), thereby better enabling locomotion. Postural aftereffects can be expected to be largest in the eye–head or hand–head systems when the near wall in on the base or apex sides, respectively.

We assessed postural adjustment contributions to prism aftereffects by comparing the magnitude of visual (eye–head) and proprioceptive (hand–head) aftereffects after subjects were instructed to walk near the wall on base or apex sides of the hallway (Redding & Wallace, 1988c). Also, aftereffects in the head–neck system were assessed by asking subjects to turn their head to be straight on their shoulders. For this test, the adaptive direction of change is in the displacement direction. Principle results are reproduced in Fig. 8.4. It should first be noted that the sum of visual and proprioceptive aftereffects (VS + PS) was not significantly different from adaptation measured by an eye–hand coordination aftereffects test (TS). Thus, there is no indication that any strategic control exercised during exposure transferred to the aftereffects tests.

Aftereffects in the head–neck system appear to be entirely postural in nature. Aftereffects appeared on this test only when the head was largely turned and not when the head was relatively straight. Possibly, this system does not include adaptive encoders for realignment. More likely, head movements in this exposure situation are not guided by specific visual position commands, but only by a more general need to center the available visual field. In any case, the fact that substantial visual eye–head aftereffects remained when head–neck aftereffects disappeared supports the assumption that the eye–head aftereffects test measures more than adaptive shift in head position. This head-relative test is sensitive to adaptive changes in position of the eyes in the head.

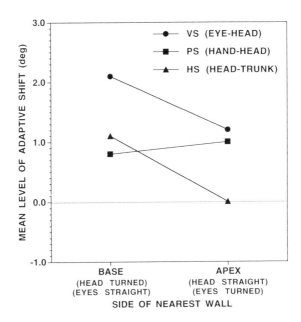

FIG. 8.4. Postural and realignment aftereffects. Adaptive shift in eye–head, hand–head, and head–neck systems as a function of differences in head and eye posture produced by walking near the hallway wall on the base or apex side of the displacing prism (data are from Redding & Wallace, 1988c).

The data also indicate that visual aftereffects are not entirely postural in nature. Aftereffects on the eye–head aftereffects test were actually larger where the least postural aftereffect of eye position was expected: that is, when the near wall was on the base side, the head was largely turned, and the eyes relatively straight in the head. Possibly, postural adjustment in eye position does occur, but clearly there is also a substantial discordance-based realignment component to adaptation in the eye–head visual system.

Finally, when subjects walked near the base-side wall, adaptive aftereffects in the hand–head system appear to be largely postural adjustments of head position. But the frequent encounters with the wall on the apex side produced adaptive realignment, probably localized in the hand–shoulder system. The hand–head aftereffects test is sensitive to all adaptive change between hand and head.

These data exclude the possibility that adaptation during locomotion consists entirely of postural adjustments. Clearly, substantial realignment also occurs. Further research is needed to assess the relative magnitude of these two kinds of adaptive change and the conditions that activate one or the other adaptive mechanism.

REALIGNMENT

Figure 8.5 summarizes what we believe happens in the case of realignment in hallway exposure. Visual guidance of locomotion is not affected by the prisms. Locomotion is guided by Gibsonlike optical flow patterns (Fitch et al., 1982; Lee & Thomson, 1982), which are little affected by the displacing prisms. Walking seems to be guided in the normal automatic manner, does not require central processing capacity, and does not suffer interference from the secondary cognitive task. The assumption of

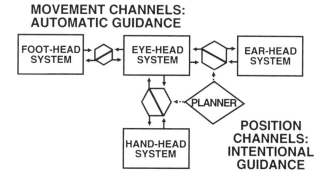

FIG. 8.5. Adaptive spatial alignment during locomotion. Locomotion is automatically guided by undistorted optical flow, whereas intentional guidance of locational responses based on distorted position is subject to interference from a secondary cognitive task, with consequential less adaptation. The manner in which the directional linkages are shown would produce adaptation in the eye–head (visual) system. From "Attention and Prism Adaptation," by G. M. Redding, S. E. Clark, and B. Wallace, 1985, *Cognitive Psychology, 17,* p. 20. Copyright 1985 by Academic Press, Inc. Reprinted with permission.

separate modules for processing motion and position information is consistent with theory construction in computational vision (e.g., Marr, 1982).

However, the continuous nature of optical flow is such that accurate locomotion can be maintained with occasional visual response to auditory or proprioceptive stimuli (Thomson, 1983). Subjects can occasionally direct their eyes to look at, for instance, another person speaking or at an obstacle they have just bumped into. On these occasions, the visual eye–head system is the guided system and local realignment occurs in this system. Such directional linkage of eye–head and ear–head or hand–head systems requires central processing capacity. When such capacity is not available because it has been allocated to mental arithmetic, these linkages occur less frequently and visual realignment decreases. Also, when visible sounding targets or proprioceptive obstacles are not present in the environment, there are no occasions for nonvisually guided looking and visual realignment will be reduced regardless of available processing capacity.

Proprioceptive realignment occurs when the direction of guidance is reversed between eye–head and hand–head systems. For instance, when subjects anticipate touching a seen obstacle, realignment tends to occur in the guided proprioceptive hand–head system. Again, such realignment of the hand–head system is reduced when capacity is not available to establish and maintain directional linkage between visual and proprioceptive systems, but the structure of the exposure task is the determinant of locus of adaptation. In the absence of auditory cues, subjects depend more heavily on proprioceptive anticipation of previously seen obstacles, thereby showing more proprioceptive realignment. Similarly, adaptation in the ear–head system may occur when, for instance, subjects turn their head to better hear a previously seen speaker. Auditory realignment is known to occur (Radeau & Bertelson, 1977, 1978), but the directionality-of-guidance explanation of this locus has not been tested.

Additional work remains to be done in hallway exposure. For example, we do not know whether the predicted auditory shifts occur in this situation. However, the determinants of visual and proprioceptive realignment are well described by our model. The most important determinant of visual realignment seems to be the ear-to-eye linkage that occurs when viewable sound sources are present. Visual aftereffects seem to be primarily discordance-based adaptation (spatial realignment) with only small contributions from asymmetric eye posture. The most important determinant of proprioceptive realignment seems to be the eye-to-hand linkage that occurs with the opportunity for proprioceptive anticipation of previously seen obstacles. Proprioceptive aftereffects also seem to be primarily discordance-based realignment with only small contributions from asymmetric head posture.

Surprisingly little evidence of strategic control has been found in our investigations of locomotion with prismatic distortion of the visual field. We might have expected such evidence to appear in failure to find additivity (VS + PS ≠ TS), reflecting transfer to the aftereffect tests of strategies deployed during exposure. The absence of such evidence may be because the primary coordination task, locomotion, is easily accomplished in uniform hallways with undistorted motion information and there is little need to deploy unusual strategies. A more substantial contribution of strategic coordination to adaptation can be expected in more complex natural environments. However, the difficulty of isolating particular adaptive contributions and the need for greater experimental control increases with increasing exposure task complexity. In our subsequent research we have, instead, turned to more artificial but experimentally controllable exposure tasks that afford the opportunity to investigate more specific predictions from the present model of prism adaptation.

SUMMARY

Locomotion in natural human environments during prism exposure is achieved by ordinary, automatic perceptual–motor control processes because optical displacement or rotation of the visual field does not distort the requisite motion information. However, orienting behaviors based on distorted positional information provide opportunities for realignment of eye–head visual or hand–head proprioceptive (and perhaps auditory) spatial systems. The locus of such realignment depends on the direction of coordinative linkage between these sensorimotor systems. Moreover, establishing and maintaining such coordinative linkages is substantially a controlled process. When resources are allocated to a secondary cognitive task, coordinative linkage does not occur, with consequent reduction in realignment aftereffects. Whereas postural adjustments in eye or head position can occur, they appear to make only minimal contributions to aftereffects obtained after hallway exploration with prismatic distortion.

Chapter 9

ADAPTIVE EYE–HAND COORDINATION

Most recently, we extended our investigation of prism adaptation to eye–hand coordination tasks. The experimental control afforded by such tasks enables a more detailed study of the component processes of adaptive perceptual–motor behavior, especially the distinction between higher level strategic control and more primitive spatial realignment. Moreover, this research paradigm connects with a larger body of work in prism adaptation (Welch, 1978, 1986) and with the question of intermittent visual control in action (Elliott, 1992; Jeannerod, 1988; Jordan & Rosenbaum, 1989; Keele, 1986).

In the first section of this chapter, we describe manipulations of visual feedback timing and movement time in eye–hand coordination, which we assume affect how the system configures coordinative linkages between spatially misaligned visual eye–head and proprioceptive hand–head subsystems. Depending on the direction and duration of coordinative linkage, differences in locus and magnitude of realignment can be predicted. Timing of online visual feedback should affect the direction of coordinative linkage with predictable change in the locus of realignment aftereffects. Movement time should also affect the locus of realignment by limiting the reversals in direction of coordinative linkage required for error evaluation and correction. However, unusually long or short movement times may disable realignment mechanisms by reducing the kinds of coordinative linkage necessary for misalignment detection and by producing a nonoptimal rate of discordance input to adaptive encoders.

In the second section, we report three sets of studies designed to identify the separate contributions of strategic control and adaptation alignment to adaptive perceptual–motor performance. In these studies, we obtain measures of performance during prism exposure as well as measures of aftereffect.

First, we tested the hypothesis that cognitive load should limit the ability to deploy controlled error-corrective strategies. To the extent that such strategies are, in part, automatic, misaligned systems may be coordinatively linked and realignment aftereffects should appear even though exposure performance may not be perfectly accurate.

Second, we distinguished between strategic control and adaptive alignment by comparing the time course of exposure aftereffects and exposure performance.

Here, the research strategy was to subtract the relatively small, slowly developing contribution of realignment aftereffects from the total adaptive response observed during exposure (direct effects). In this manner, we derive an estimate of the larger, more rapidly developing contribution from strategic control. We were able to identify several control strategies, not all of which are conducive to realignment.

Third, we tested the hypothesis that realignment depends on comparison of achieved limb position with the expected limb position supplied by the feedforward calibration signal. These studies are also a test of the assumption that feedforward and feedback control involve distinct control signals based on position and difference codes, respectively.

METHODOLOGY

Our model assumes that coordinative linkage is strategically dependent on the structure of the coordination task and that the locus of discordance detection and realignment is hierarchically subordinate to the configuration of coordinative linkages. For this reason it is important to specify, as exactly as present knowledge permits, the relevant characteristics of the prism exposure task.

The following experiments employed a paced, reciprocal-movement, target-pointing task, usually in the sagittal dimension, performed under 11.4 deg (20 diopters) optical displacement in the rightward direction. The limited visual field imposed by prism-bearing goggles commonly prevented view of the limb in the starting position and for approximately the first half of the pointing movement. Secondary corrections, after the primary movement had been completed, were discouraged and appeared only infrequently.

Pointing movements were made in time to a metronome signal and were most often unconstrained by surface contacts during or at the terminal end of the movement. In most experiments, subjects were instructed to initiate a movement on one beat, move the limb such that it was fully extended on the next beat, withdraw the limb such that the hand arrived back at the starting position on the third beat, and so on. In this manner, a smooth movement cycle was achieved for every three beats of the metronome with minimal hesitation on a beat and relatively constant velocity between beats. Typically, movements were relatively slow (e.g., with the metronome set to beat every 3 s) and few in number (e.g., 60).

When exposure performance was assessed, terminal error between the pointing finger and the target was measured. These observations were made when the subject's finger paused briefly, signaling primary movement completion and before any secondary movement. Because secondary movements were discouraged, the use of visual feedback was almost entirely restricted to online control of the primary movement. Little use was made of visual feedback to initiate secondary corrections after the primary movement had been completed. Of course, visual information about terminal error (knowledge of results) on a previous trial could be used to initiate the primary movement on the next trial.

Aftereffect measures of spatial realignment in the eye–head visual system and the hand–head proprioceptive system were obtained. For the visual shift (VS) test, subjects were instructed to adjust (usually by verbal instructions to the experimenter) a visual target to appear straight ahead of the nose without error feedback or knowledge of results. For the proprioceptive shift (PS) test, subjects were instructed to point straight ahead of the nose without sight of the hand or knowledge of results. These measures were obtained both before and after prism exposure. The pretest provided baselines from which change in posttests could be assessed.

Because the VS and PS tests are referenced to the head, comparisons of performance on these tests before and after prism exposure provide measures of adaptive change in the eye–head and hand–head systems, respectively. Moreover, because these aftereffect tests are performed without error feedback or knowledge of results and subjects were informed that the prismatic distortion was not present, they are arguably measures of realignment rather than of strategic control (see also chapters 4 and 7).

A total shift (TS) aftereffect measure was obtained by having subjects point at a visual target before and after prism exposure without sight of their limb or knowledge of results. The inclusion of this measure enabled the additivity test (VS + PS = TS). Because the TS test is sensitive to any adaptive change in systems inclusive of eye and hand, deviation from additivity can be taken as an indicator of adaptive strategies deployed during prism exposure which transfer to the aftereffect tests.

COORDINATIVE LINKAGE

A central problem in motor control theory is the development of a reasoned account of the variety of ways in which a coordinated response can be achieved.[1] From the current perspective, one aspect of this problem is the nature of coordinative linkage between component sensorimotor systems. Depending on how eye and hand are coordinatively linked, the locus and magnitude of realignment vary (chapter 6). If coordinative linkage is eye-to-hand, realignment is visual in nature, but if the linkage is hand-to-eye the realignment is localized in the proprioceptive hand–head system. If the linkage is strategically mediated, realignment of any kind will be reduced and may not occur at all (chapter 5).

Although realignment is assumed to be mandatory (automatic), it is largely dependent on higher level coordination processes to establish the necessary conditions for discordance detection and realignment. In this section, we review manipulations that affect coordinative linkage of eye and hand with predictable indirect effects on realignment.

Visual Feedback Timing

In a fundamental sense, visual feedback must be available, or spatial discordance cannot be detected, and realignment cannot occur. Without such sensory feedback,

---

[1]See also the discussion of the Degrees-of-Freedom Problem in chapter 1.

achieved position will not be available for comparison with expected position and the discordance signal for realignment will not occur (chapter 6). Thus, the absence of visual feedback makes the uninteresting prediction of no spatial realignment. However, the point in time during coordinated action of eyes and hand when visual feedback is available will determine the direction of coordinative linkage, with predictable consequences for the locus of realignment aftereffects.

Sight of the limb early in a pointing movement should encourage an overall visual guidance strategy. For example, the knowledge that a view of the limb will be available for comparison with the visual target, thereby enabling possible in-flight correction, should encourage selection of the visual target for initiation of both eye and hand actions. With such eye-to-hand coordinative linkage, misalignment detection and realignment will occur in the proprioceptive hand–head system.

Delaying sight of the limb until later in the pointing movement decreases the possibility of visually based correction, thereby encouraging reliance on proprioceptive information from the limb to set the target for eye and hand. Such hand-to-eye coordinative linkage will localize misalignment detection and realignment in the visual eye–head system. Moreover, given that visual feedback is available at some point in the movement, discordance should have the same magnitude, no matter whether it occurs in the visual or proprioceptive system. Thus, the timing of visual feedback should have its effects in determining the direction of coordinative linkage between misaligned systems and consequently on the locus of realignment. The timing of visual feedback availability should have no role in determining the total amount of realignment.

Several early studies support these predictions (Cohen, 1967; Freedman, 1968; Uhlarik & Canon, 1971). Redding and Wallace (1988b) firmly established the predicted reciprocal relationship in magnitude of visual and proprioceptive realignment aftereffects for early and late visual feedback over a variety of exposure conditions. We have further shown a graded effect, such that as sight of the pointing limb was increasingly delayed, proprioceptive realignment decreased while visual realignment increased (Redding & Wallace, 1988a).

In all of these studies, however, continuous view of the pointing limb was available beyond the time in the pointing movement where the limb first become visible. Duration of visual feedback (how much of the movement enjoyed visual feedback) and timing of visual feedback (when feedback became available in the course of a pointing movement) were confounded. An extended view of the moving limb may enable more visual correction and better achievement of the target, but should not change the eye-to-hand linkage already induced by early visual feedback. Moreover, in-flight correction is assumed to be based on difference signals and should not affect misalignment detection and realignment based on position signals (chapters 5 and 6). From the present theoretical perspective, timing of visual feedback should be more important than duration of visual feedback in determining the locus of realignment.

Redding and Wallace (1990) separated the effects of duration and timing of visual feedback. In Experiment 2, for example, the available visual field (approximately 25 cm in the sagittal dimension) was occluded to permit a 2.5 cm view of the fingertip with the pointing limb fully extended. Then, the time in the pointing movement at which sight of the limb first became available was manipulated by introducing a 2.5 cm gap in the occluder. This gap was centered at increasing distances from the beginning of the available visual field. The duration of visual feedback was constant whereas the time at which visual feedback first became available varied from early to late in the pointing movement.

For each of these conditions, different groups of subjects engaged in 60 reciprocal movements (movement distance approximately 50 cm), pointing toward the position in space believed to be straight ahead of the nose with approximately 1.5 s for each outward or backward movement segment, and with their visual field displaced 11.4 deg (20 diopters) in the rightward direction. Results are illustrated in Fig. 9.1.

As in previous studies, additivity was nearly perfect (Redding & Wallace, 1988a, 1988b). The average total adaptive shift (TS) in the eye–hand system (3.9 deg) was

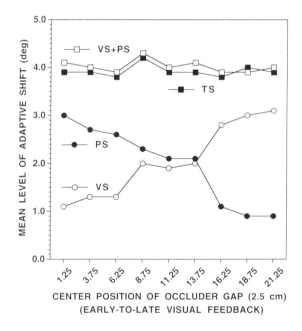

FIG. 9.1. Visual feedback timing and realignment. Adaptive shift in the visual eye–head (VS) and proprioceptive hand–head (PS) systems as a function of the time in the pointing movement when the limb first became visible. When the limb first became visible was manipulated by varying the position in the available visual field (25 cm) of a 2.5 cm gap in an occluding shelf. Also shown are the sum of visual and proprioceptive shifts (VS + PS) and the total adaptive shift in the eye–hand system (TS). (Data from Redding & Wallace, 1990, Experiment 2.) Reprinted from G. M. Redding and B. Wallace, "Adaptive Eye–Hand Coordination: Implications of Prism Adaptation for Perceptual Motor Control." In L. Proteau and D. Elliot (Eds.), *Vision and Motor Control,* Copyright 1992, p. 109, by Elsevier Science—NL, Sara Burgerhartstraat 25, 1055 KV Amsterdam, The Netherlands.

almost exactly the same as the average sum of adaptive shifts (VS + PS) in the visual eye–head and proprioceptive hand–head systems (4.0 deg). Moreover, by either measure, the timing of visual feedback (delay in gap occurrence) affected the locus, but not the total amount of realignment.

As can be seen in Fig. 9.1, aftereffects in the visual eye–head system (VS) increased with increasing delay in the time during movement at which visual feedback was first available. This result is consistent with the prediction that when visual feedback is not available early in a pointing movement, subjects strategically activate hand-to-eye coordinative linkage and realignment is therefore localized in the visual system.

Also as predicted from decreasing ability to rely on visual guidance (eye-to-hand linkage), realignment aftereffects in the proprioceptive hand–head system (PS) decreased with visual feedback delay. Unlike the nearly linear change in VS, however, PS showed an additional abrupt change when view of the limb was delayed beyond 13.75 cm. Assuming that average limb length is about 50 cm, with the first 25 cm occluded by the prism-bearing goggles, the sharp decrease in PS occurred when visual feedback was delayed beyond about 38 cm, or three fourths of the way to the terminal position.

These results suggest that visual feedback is utilized early in the course of a pointing movement to guide both hand and eye, with consequent eye-to-hand coordinative linkage and realignment in the guided hand–head system. As visual feedback is delayed until later in the pointing movement, it becomes increasingly more difficult to utilize the information until, about three fourths of the way to the terminal position, it becomes abruptly unusable. It may be that the limb is ballistically released at this point and is no longer under feedback control. Alternatively, limb position made available by previous hand-to-eye linkage might be used to activate feedforward control based on the difference between limb and target.[2] In any case, as visual feedback becomes less usable, proprioceptive feedback may be utilized to guide both eye and hand, with consequent hand-to-eye coordinative linkage and realignment in the guided eye–head system.

This view of movement control is strikingly different from the traditional view of intermittent control of reaching or aiming movements (Keele, 1981; Paillard, 1982; see also chapter 1). Accurate aiming movements are commonly observed to include an initial high-velocity, presumably feedforward control, component and a terminal low-velocity component during which visual feedback may be utilized to make trajectory corrections.[3]

The use of visual feedback earlier rather than later in a movement may depend on the absence of surface contacts in the present method. A natural tendency to slow movement when approaching an impending surface contact could account for the terminal low-velocity component in many reaching or aiming studies, and the

---

[2]But see chapter 5 for arguments against the use of difference codes in feedforward control.

[3]Although this description is commonly accepted (e.g., Annett, Golby, & Kay, 1958; Beggs & Howarth, 1972; Woodworth, 1899), some recent investigations question its generality (Elliott, 1992; Goodale, Pélisson, & Prablanc, 1986; Jeannerod, 1984).

diminishing of movement velocity could better enable utilization of visual feedback in the final stages of movement. In the absence of surface contacts, movement velocity may actually increase in later movement phases and visual feedback may be more useful during low-velocity initial phases. Movements involving surface contact may, therefore, be kinematically different from the present movements, involving different patterns of change in the direction of coordinative linkage with consequent differences in locus of realignment aftereffects.

In any case, the present data clearly support the prediction that timing of visual feedback affects the kind, but not the total amount of realignment. This result is consistent with the present view that visual feedback affects the temporal pattern of coordinative linkage among component systems to optimize performance, but does not directly affect realignment. Delaying sight of the pointing limb may modify coordinative linkage routines for identifying the source of performance error (chapter 7). A focus on correcting limb movements (visual guidance) may shift to a predominant concern with correcting eye movement (proprioceptive guidance), with consequential shift in the locus of realignment from the hand–head system to the eye–head system.

Movement Time

Several features of the present model suggest that the length of the interval between onset and termination of the pointing movement (movement time) should be a relevant variable for realignment. For instance, changes in coordinative linkage between eye and hand to identify the source of performance error (chapter 7) may be strategically dependent on movement time. As shown in the preceding section, with very long movement times on the order of about 1.5 s or more, directional changes in linkage are possible. In such cases, depending on visual feedback delay, the relative proportion of eye-to-hand and hand-to-eye linkage determines the locus, but not the total amount of realignment.

For shorter movement times, error-evaluation routines may become more difficult. Actual reversal of coordinative linkage (hand-to-eye) should eventually become impossible, with consequent loss of eye–head realignment. In-flight correction based on purely visual error evaluation (exclusive eye-to-hand linkage) should remain possible for somewhat shorter movement times, but with very short movement times, difference-coded commands to reduce error should become impossible to calculate and even hand–head (proprioceptor) realignment should disappear. Performance error can still be reduced even for rapid movements by knowledge of results compensation applied over successive trials, but such mediated linkage of eye and hand removes the stimulus for realignment (chapters 5 and 6). The expectation is that realignment should decrease with decreasing movement time, more quickly for eye–head than for head–hand realignment.

Note that movement time rather than movement speed seems to be the more important variable. A constant, long-duration movement over short and long distances may allow sufficient time for both error evaluation and feedback correction, even though the two movements are different in speed. Mechanical constraints (e.g., inertia) make movement speed crucial for the performance of very rapid movements that require predictive feedforward control. However, feedforward control and the rapid error correction it affords is not possible in the present situation because the naive subject does not have available movement plans that can anticipate the prismatic displacement (chapter 1).[4] Moreover, long before speed becomes important, movement time may become too short to permit the processes of strategic control necessary for realignment.

The predicted effects of movement time on locus and magnitude of realignment may be mitigated by the spacing of pointing movements (distribution of practice). Error evaluation and correction could occur between movements after the primary movement is completed but while the limb is visible and visual feedback is still available. The reversal in directional linkage associated with error evaluation could produce discordance detection and realignment in the eye–head system. Corrective changes in hand position to achieve the target should produce discordance and realignment in the hand–head system. Distributed practice with rest periods imposed between pointing movements should facilitate realignment even if actual movement time is short, especially if the hand remains in view and is not withdrawn immediately after completion of the primary movement.

Confounding of intermovement interval and movement time may be responsible for the contradictory results from studies of distribution of practice effects in prism adaptation (for reviews, see Welch, 1978, 1986). The following experiments isolated effects of movement time on realignment by holding the intermovement interval constant (see the previous Methodology section), thereby minimizing confounding from error evaluation and correction after completion of the primary movement.

A factor complicating interpretation of movement time effects is the response rate of adaptive encoders (chapter 7). As movement time is decreased without pause between movements, the rate of discordance input increases. Effects of movement time may, therefore, be confused with limits on the ability of encoders to respond to discordance signals.

One way to separate movement time and input rate effects may be to obtain measures of the growth of realignment over successive pointing trials. Movement time is assumed to affect the duration of coordinative linkages and consequently the amount of realignment. However, once a linkage between misaligned systems has been established, for whatever duration, the rate at which realignment develops over successive movements should depend on the operational parameters of the adaptive encoder in the guided system. Thus, movement time can be expected to have distinct effects on the asymptotic amount of realignment and the rate at which realignment approaches that limit.

Long movement times and low discordance-input rates less than the time constant of an encoder should permit decay of realignment, whereas short movement times and high discordance-input rates greater than the time constant of an encoder should overdrive the realignment mechanism. And the optimal input rate

---

[4]Associative learning of a movement plan appropriate for the prismatic displacement is possible, but this removes the stimulus for realignment (chapter 5).

may be expected to be different for different encoders with different time constants. Deviation from optimal input rate in either direction should slow the growth of realignment. There should, then, be a range of movement times that produces the same rates of growth in realignment, although different for the different sensorimotor systems. Within this range, however, decreasing movement time should still produce the predicted decrease in amount of realignment.

Movement time effects may also be confused with effects of visual feedback timing. As movement time decreases, visual feedback becomes increasingly less useful and the situation would seem to approach that of extreme delay of feedback. However, the predicted effects of such decreased utilization of feedback are quite different from those of feedback delay. Shorter movement times decrease the ability to engage in error evaluation and correction involving hand-to-eye linkage and increase reliance on unidirectional eye-to-hand linkage. Thus, shorter movement times should produce more realignment in the hand–head system than in the eye–head system, regardless of feedback availability. Separating the effects of movement time and feedback delay, therefore, requires orthogonal manipulation of the two variables.

Partial confirmation of these predictions has been obtained by assessing the growth of realignment aftereffects in the eye–head and hand–head systems under conditions defined by orthogonal combinations of movement time and feedback delay (Redding & Wallace, 1992b, 1994). Movement time was manipulated by setting the paced pointing (reciprocal sagittal movements) at levels of one complete out and back sagittal pointing movement every 1, 2, 3, 4, or 6 s. Because the pause at either (initiation or termination) end of the movement was small, movement times were approximately .5, 1.0, 1.5, 2.0, or 3.0 s for these pointing rates.

Visual feedback timing was manipulated by restricting sight of the limb to the last joint of the pointing index finger (late feedback) or the hand to mid-forearm (early feedback) when the limb was in the fully extended position.[5] Aftereffect measures of eye–head realignment or visual shift (VS) and hand–head realignment or proprioceptive shift (PS) were obtained after blocks of 10 pointing trials, performed with 11.4 deg rightward optical displacement of the visual field.

These manipulations were performed in a series of two published experiments (Redding & Wallace, 1992b, 1994) and one previously unreported experiment. Several differences among the three experiments should be mentioned. Redding and Wallace (1994) tested movement times of .5, 1.5, and 3.0 s, with 80 exposure trials of pointing toward an objectively straight-ahead target. Redding and Wallace (1992b) tested movement times of 1.0 and 1.5 s, with 60 exposure trials pointing toward the position in space believed to be straight ahead of the nose. The previously unreported experiment was similar to Redding and Wallace (1992b), except that movement times of 1.5 and 2 s were tested. Only the data for the first 60 trials from Redding and Wallace (1994) were included in the present analysis. Despite these differences among experiments, the data present a consistent pattern.

---

[5]These late and early feedback conditions correspond to what are sometimes called *terminal* and *concurrent feedback,* respectively (e.g., Redding & Wallace, 1990; Uhlarik & Canon, 1971).

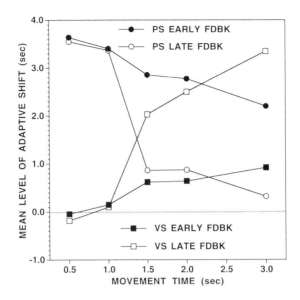

FIG. 9.2. Movement time, visual feedback timing, and realignment. Adaptive shift in the visual eye–head (VS) and proprioceptive hand–head (PS) systems as function of duration of the sagittal pointing movement (Movement Time). Data are also shown for early visual feedback in which most of the limb was visible in the fully extended position and late visual feedback in which only the last joint of the pointing finger was visible (data from Redding & Wallace, 1992b, 1994, and a previously unreported study).

Figure 9.2 illustrates the different effects of feedback delay and movement time on the locus of realignment when the data were averaged over blocks of exposure trials. With slow movements of 1.5 s or longer, the usual reciprocal effect of early versus late visual feedback on VS and PS appeared (Redding & Wallace, 1988b; Uhlarik & Canon, 1971). This result is consistent with the assumption that delay of feedback until the end of a pointing movement causes a strategic shift from largely visual to more proprioceptive guidance. With faster movements of 1.0 s or less, there was no effect of feedback delay on the locus of realignment, but VS decreased accompanied by a corresponding increase in PS. When insufficient time is available for in-flight error evaluation, the hand-to-eye reversal in coordinative linkage does not occur and task performance involves solely eye-to-hand linkage. These results clearly demonstrate the distinct effects of feedback delay and movement time on realignment.

The expected decrease in both visual and proprioceptive realignment aftereffects did not appear at the shortest movement time tested. Visual eye–head realignment clearly decreased to zero with a movement time of .5 s, but proprioceptive hand–head realignment continued to increase. This movement time, however, is still long compared to common practice in motor control research. We expect that with such shorter movement times purely visual error evaluation and correction should become increasingly more difficult, direct coordinative linkage between systems should decrease in frequency, and even hand–head realignment will decrease and eventually disappear.

The pattern of effects displayed in Fig. 9.2 were consistent over all trial blocks and the growth of realignment components over trial blocks was differentially affected only by movement time. This result supports the assumption that growth rate provides a measure of encoder response rate distinct from factors affecting the direction and duration of coordinative linkage.

The differential effect of movement time on growth of visual and proprioceptive realignment is illustrated in Fig. 9.3. If we assume that the asymptotic limits of these growth functions reflect the proportions of proprioceptive and visual guidance, then the different rates at which the functions approach their limits provide measures of the response rate of visual and proprioceptive encoders.

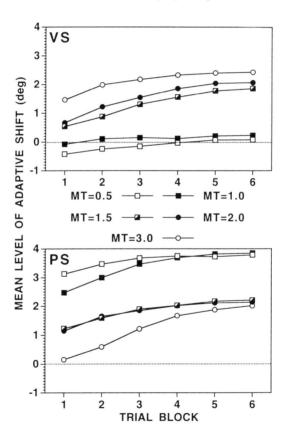

FIG. 9.3. Movement time and growth of realignment. Adaptive shift in the visual eye–head (VS) and proprioceptive hand–head (PS) systems as function of blocks of 10 exposure pointing trials with different movement times (MT) for the sagittal pointing movement (data from Redding & Wallace, 1992b, 1994, and a previously unreported study).

Growth of visual eye–head realignment (VS) is clearly favored by the longer movement times, whereas realignment in the proprioceptive hand–head systems (PS) increases more rapidly with shorter movement times. The nearly zero growth of VS with the shorter movement times (.5 and 1.0 s) may reflect an inability of the visual encoder to keep pace with successive discordance inputs. The 1.5 and 2.0 s movement times seem to overdrive the visual encoder to a lesser degree and the nearly asymptotic VS for the 3.0 s movement time after the first block of trials suggest that this may be near the optimal input rate. Movement time much longer than 3.0 s should permit decay of realignment with consequent decrease in rate of growth for visual realignment aftereffects.

On the other hand, the 3.0 s movement time appears to permit substantial decay of proprioceptive realignment (PS). Movement times of 2.0 and 1.5 s allow less decay and the 1.0 s movement time involves even less decay of proprioceptive realignment. The observation that PS does not reach an early asymptote for the .5 s movement time suggests that the optimal input rate may be afforded by a still shorter movement time. Further manipulation of movement time should enable better estimation of the operational parameters of adaptive encoders.

These results suggest that the short movement times typical of most research in motor control may disable adaptive alignment mechanisms. Some other evidence is available that realignment requires comparatively slow movements. Smith and Bowen (1980) found that performance during prism exposure increased for increases in movement time up to about 650 ms, with some indication of further improvement if longer times had been used. To the extent that exposure performance is mediated in part by realignment, not just strategic control, these observations suggest that realignment requires long movement times.

Baily (1972) argued that realignment, as opposed to strategic control, occurred for very long movement times of about 6.25 s, but not for short movement times of about 220 ms. Movement times on the order of 250 ms or more may be needed for realignment of any kind to occur. Performance during prism exposure with very short movement times may depend largely on more deliberate coordination strategies such as knowledge-of-results compensation (chapter 7).

STRATEGIC CONTROL

The assumption that adaptive alignment mechanisms are hierarchically subordinate to coordination strategies poses a special methodological problem. Because misalignment detection and realignment depends on coordinative linkage of misaligned systems, any manipulation that precludes such linkage should also preclude realignment. It becomes difficult, therefore, to assess the separate contributions of these two adaptive processes to overall adaptive behavior.

In this section, we present the results from three sets of studies that manipulated the separate contributions of strategic control and adaptive alignment. The first set of studies examined the effect of cognitive load on realignment aftereffects and performance during prism exposure. These experiments tested the assumption of differential involvement of higher level, capacity-limited processes in the two kinds of adaptation. The second set of studies more directly tested the assumed distinct kinds of adaptation by a more extensive comparison of performance during prism exposure direct effects with aftereffect measures of realignment. Also in these studies, manipulations of visual feedback delay and target uncertainty were introduced to assess differential effects on the two kinds of adaptation.

The third set of studies tested the hypothesis that realignment is dependent on comparison of achieved limb position with the expected limb position supplied by the feedforward calibration signal. This test compared an exposure condition likely to involve only feedback control that should not produce realignment, with the usual exposure condition that is known to produce realignment.

Cognitive Load

In the present model, adaptive alignment is a low-level primitive process that is automatically activated whenever misalignment between parts of the perceptual–motor system is detected. In contrast, strategic control is a higher level process that can be influenced by controlled processes that, for example, interpret the task-relevance of error feedback. Controlled processes are conceived of as more deliberate, slow, monitored processes that draw on limited central processing capacity. Automatic processes are more habitual, fast routines that have less or perhaps no capacity limitation. If this distinction between automatic and controlled processes is valid, then realignment should be less affected than strategic control by a secondary task that imposes a cognitive load.

A complicating factor for this hypothesis is the assumption that coordination and alignment mechanisms are hierarchically related. Alignment mechanisms reside in subcomponents of the perceptual–motor system, below the level of coordinative linkage between components. The implication of this hierarchical arrangement is that misaligned systems must be coordinatively linked in order for the misalignment to be detected and for realignment to occur. Realignment is the automatic response to spatial discordance, but discordance detection depends on higher level coordination processes. Thus, interference with coordination can also indirectly interfere with realignment (Redding et al., 1985; see also chapter 8).

A possible resolution of this dilemma lies in the recognition that, depending on the level of analysis, automatic versus controlled processing is not a dichotomous distinction. At a molecular level of analysis, parts of a process may be controlled whereas other parts are automatic (Shiffrin & Dumais, 1981; see also chapters 1, 7, and 8). Eye–hand coordination is surely such a multipart process.

In particular, for some kinds of tasks, eye–hand coordinative linkage may be activated automatically, but further utilization of feedback to fine tune the action may require more controlled processing. It may be possible to find an eye–hand coordination task that includes enough controlled processing to show cognitive load effects on exposure performance but that is also sufficiently automatic to assure coordinative linkage and consequent substantial realignment. The absence of substantial effects on realignment aftereffects in the presence of significant effects on exposure performance would constitute clear evidence of distinct mechanisms for adaptive alignment and strategic control.

This was the research strategy followed by Redding et al., (1992). The primary task was paced (2 s rate) sagittal target pointing under optical displacement with visual feedback available early in the pointing movement. As previously noted, this task evokes primarily visual guidance, especially when pointing movements are made rapidly (Redding & Wallace, 1988a, 1988b, 1990, 1992b). Such visual guidance meets the criterion of an habitual, fast process and should enable sufficiently automatic coordinative linkage for misalignment detection and re-alignment to occur.

Nevertheless, the pointing task was expected to include sufficient controlled processing, such as error evaluation and correction, so that fine tuning of exposure performance should show interference from the cognitive load imposed by the secondary task. The secondary cognitive task was mental arithmetic, which previous research showed to be demanding of the central processing capacity required for controlled coordinative linkage (Redding et al., 1985; Redding & Wallace, 1985a, 1985b; see also chapter 8). Strategic control was assessed by terminal error on the primary task and adaptive alignment by aftereffect measures.

In two experiments, cognitive load was found to have a small, but significant effect on primary task performance and little or no effect on aftereffect measures. For instance, in Experiment 2, terminal pointing error during prism exposure averaged near zero over the 60 trials at .2 deg in the displacement direction without cognitive load. With cognitive load, terminal error was significantly greater than zero at 1.5 deg in the displacement direction. In contrast, the aftereffect measure of total realignment in the eye–hand system (TS) was nonsignificantly greater with mental arithmetic (3.0 deg) compared to no secondary task (2.9 deg). Performance on the secondary task supported the assumption that mental arithmetic did, in fact, impose cognitive load. Subjects successfully solved an average of only about 74% of the slightly more than 20 problems attempted, with a new problem being received on average about once every 6 s.

These results suggest that cognitive load disables the normal error evaluation and correction routines needed to maximize performance. For instance, the momentary reversal of coordinative linkage required for determining the source of an error (chapter 7) may be a more controlled process and largely not possible when central processing capacity is otherwise occupied. Consistent with this interpretation was a tendency for realignment in the eye–head system (VS) to be reduced under cognitive load, although the level of such visual shift was too low to permit a reliable conclusion (see also Rader, 1989). Subjects may fall back on more automatic visual guidance with consequential inability to correct the residual performance error arising from the displacement. At a more phenomenal level of description, with attention directed toward the arithmetic problems, subjects may simply accept small performance errors (Proteau, 1992).

Aftereffects and Direct Effects

If strategic control and adaptive alignment are distinct but hierarchically organized processes, both kinds of processes should contribute to adaptive performance during exposure to an optically induced misalignment. That is, the large performance error produced by misalignment should activate coordination strategies for error reduction and spatial discordance between coordinatively linked systems should produce local realignment. Direct effect measures of performance change during exposure to misalignment should reflect the joint contributions of strategic control and adaptive alignment.

In contrast, when the misalignment is removed (i.e., postexposure) and information about performance error is eliminated, change in performance should reflect only persistence of adaptive change in alignment. If the subject knows that the optical distortion has been removed and information about performance error is not available, there is no basis for development of error-reduction strategies and no reason to assume continued application of such coordination strategies acquired during exposure to the misalignment. Aftereffect measures of performance relative to baseline should provide a relatively pure measure of realignment without contamination from coordination strategies (see also chapter 4).

The comparison of aftereffects and direct effects is a research strategy for identifying the separate contributions of strategic control and adaptive alignment to adaptive behavior. Aftereffects are more or less direct measures of realignment and the difference between direct effects and aftereffects provides an indirect measure of coordination strategies.

Consistent with this interpretation is the usually observed, but infrequently reported, greater compensation during exposure, compared to after exposure to optical misalignment (e.g., Baily, 1972). The magnitude of direct effects that include both adaptive alignment and strategic coordination should be greater than aftereffects that measure only adaptive alignment. Moreover, the growth over the exposure period of direct effects that include contribution from short-term error-reduction strategies should be faster than the growth of aftereffects that include only long-term realignment.

Redding and Wallace (1993) applied this research strategy. Terminal error direct effects were measured on each of 60 paced sagittal target-pointing trials paced at a 3 s rate with visual and proprioceptive aftereffects measured after each block of 10 trials. In addition, visual feedback delay and target uncertainty were manipulated to assess differential effects on the two kinds of adaptation. In separate experiments, subjects pointed at an implicit "straight-ahead-of-the-nose" target or an explicit objectively straight-ahead target. In each experiment, visual feedback was available either early in the pointing movement or delayed until the end of the movement.

To facilitate comparison of contributions from strategic control and adaptive alignment, results are expressed in Fig. 9.4 as percentage compensation for the 11.4 deg rightward optical displacement. These data represent the terminal error relative to objective target position for every 10th exposure trial and the sum of the immediately following visual shift and proprioceptive shift aftereffect tests.

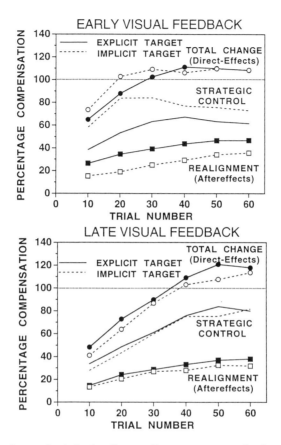

FIG. 9.4.   Strategic control and adaptive alignment. Percentage compensation for misalignment as a function of trial number for early and late visual feedback conditions with an explicit (objectively straight-ahead) target and an implicit (straight-ahead-of-the-nose) target. Total change reflects the direct effects on terminal error for every 10th exposure trial expressed as percent of the 11.4 deg optical displacement. Realignment reflects the sum of aftereffects in the eye–head and hand–head systems following each block of 10 exposure trials expressed as percent of optical displacement. The difference between direct effects and aftereffects is also displayed as an estimate of the strategic control contribution to adaptive performance (data from Redding & Wallace, 1993).

The most salient feature of these data is that direct effect measures of total adaptive change rapidly achieved complete compensation for the misalignment early in exposure. Aftereffect measures of realignment more slowly achieved levels of only about 30% to 40% compensation by the end of the exposure period. The strategic control contribution, estimated by the difference between direct effects and aftereffects, was substantially larger that the realignment contribution. The estimate of strategic control achieved levels of 70% to 80% compensation by the end of exposure. In fact, the joint contribution of strategic control and adaptive alignment (direct effects) showed about 10% to 20% overcompensation for the misalignment, although there was a tendency toward reduction of this overcompensation toward the end of exposure.

With delayed visual feedback, strategic control and overcompensation developed more slowly, but achieved a higher level, compared to early visual feedback. Whether the target was explicit or implicit made little difference when feedback was delayed. With early visual feedback, however, the explicit target produced greater realignment and less strategic control. The clearest tendency was a reduction of the overcompensation toward the end of the exposure period. This pattern of results suggests a complicated and not always cooperative interaction of strategic control and adaptive alignment.

More specifically, results with delayed feedback suggest a coordination strategy that slowly compensates for performance error arising from the misalignment. This strategy is difficult to modify when overcompensation occurs and is applicable with both explicit and implicit targets. Delay in visual feedback may encourage dependence on continuously available proprioceptive feedback and selection of a target position in hand–head space for the coordinated action of both eyes and hand. Such hand-to-eye coordinative linkage is indicated by the fact that the larger part of realignment was visual in nature when visual feedback was delayed with both explicit and implicit targets.

The strategic coordination component may arise from adoption of a successive-approximations error-reduction strategy. Over successive trials, subjects shift the proprioceptive target in relatively small steps such that when the limb becomes visible, it appears successively closer to the visually coded target position. In this manner the gradual error-reduction shown in Fig. 9.4 develops. When the finger becomes visible, the misalignment-produced discrepancy between seen position and expected position, based on visual expression of proprioceptive coordinates, constitutes locally detected discordance and motivates realignment of the visual exteroceptor.

If, in the likely case that a corrective saccade is made to fixate the finger, misalignment detection and reduction would shift to the visual proprioceptor. But in either case, the locus of realignment would be the eye–head system (chapter 6). Such successive approximation may require several trials before resetting can be achieved, especially when a reversal in direction of movement is required. As realignment gradually develops, the resultant target overshooting (overcompensation) is slow to be corrected.

In contrast, results with early visual feedback suggest different coordination strategies for explicit and implicit targets. These strategies more rapidly compensate for performance error arising from misalignment and are more readily modified when overcompensation occurs. Early visual feedback encourages visual guidance; selection of a visual target for coordinated action of eyes and hand. Such eye-to-hand coordinative linkage is indicated by the fact that the larger part of realignment occurred in the hand–head system with early visual feedback for both explicit and implicit targets.

An explicit target may permit online adjustment in limb trajectory, zeroing-out the difference between seen target position and seen hand position (Jakobson & Goodale, 1989). Such feedback control by difference-coded signals would leave intact the original position signal that initiated movement. This provides a basis for discordance between achieved position of the limb and expected position based on proprioceptive expression of visual coordinates with consequential realignment in the hand–head system. A zeroing-out strategy would enable large adjustments in pointing, with consequential rapid target achievement and better correction for overshooting that arises as realignment develops.

A zeroing-out strategy is more difficult to apply in the absence of an explicit target. Rather, with only an implicit target subjects depend more on a side-pointing strategy, selecting as the target for pointing a visual position to the side of where straight-ahead-of-the-nose looks to be, so that the pointing limb appears on target at the end of the movement. Within precision limits, the limb achieves the commanded position, the achieved hand position agrees with the expected position based on proprioceptively expressed visual coordinates, and there is no discordance basis for realignment in the hand–head system.

Substantial dependence on a side-pointing strategy may, therefore, be responsible for the lower level of realignment obtained for the implicit target compared to the explicit target with early visual feedback (see Fig. 9.4). Such side-pointing enables large adjustments in pointing, with rapid target achievement. However, correction for past-pointing (overcompensation) as realignment develops is slow because of difficulty in resetting between pointing movements. Several trials may be necessary before a new side target can be selected.

Comparison of direct effects and aftereffects offers an heuristic method for investigating the joint effects of strategic control and adaptive alignment on adaptive performance. Indeed, interpretation of differences between these two kinds of measures depends on recognition of these distinct contributions to adaptation. Failure to recognize these separate sources of adaptation may be the basis for the unfortunate tendency for researchers to extract only one or the other kind of measure.

Researchers with a primary theoretical interest in strategic control tend to focus on performance during prism exposure (direct effects) and are puzzled by reports of contrasting low levels of adaptation revealed by aftereffects measures. Researchers whose interest is in understanding adaptive alignment look primarily at aftereffects and are equally puzzled by the near perfect performance observed during prism exposure. The present theoretical framework offers the means to a better understanding of the multiple sources of adaptive perceptual–motor behavior.

Feedforward and Feedback Control

Feedforward and feedback control are the two general kinds of strategies available to the perceptual–motor system (chapter 1). We argued in chapter 5 that feedforward and feedback control ordinarily involve distinct kinds of control signals that code position and differences between positions, respectively.

We hypothesized that, only if a pointing movement is initiated in a feedforward manner with the position of a visual target, can the targeted position for common action of eyes and hand be preserved as a calibration signal for comparison with achieved position of the limb. And such a comparison is necessary for misalignment detection (chapter 6).[6] Subsequent feedback control, after movement initiation, utilizes difference codes and does not alter the initiating position code. A prediction from this view of feedforward and feedback control is that if a pointing movement is performed solely under feedback control, realignment aftereffects will not appear, even though feedback control may enable near perfect performance during prism exposure.

We have now confirmed this prediction several times with both lateral (Redding & Wallace, 1996a) and sagittal (Redding & Wallace, 1996b) pointing movements, and with both reciprocal (Redding & Wallace, 1995a) and discrete (Redding & Wallace, 1996b) movements. Our research strategy has been to compare experimental and control conditions of exposure to prismatic displacement. In the experimental condition, the starting position for a movement and the target position were simultaneously visible. In the control condition only the target position was visible.

For example, Redding and Wallace (1995a) had subjects make 30 sagittal pointing movements from a tactile starting position toward a visible target at a rate of 1 out-and-back movement every 3 s producing a movement time approximately 1.5 s. The visual field was optically displaced 11.4 deg (20 diopters) in the rightward direction. For the control condition (nonvisible starting position), the starting position was occluded by a black cloth. For the experimental condition (visible starting position), the occluding cloth was removed. Exposure performance in pointing at the visible target was recorded for each trial and aftereffects were assessed by measures obtained before and after the 30 pointing trials. The results of this experiment are displayed in Fig. 9.5.

For the nonvisible starting position group, accurate performance during exposure was slow to develop, even though substantial realignment aftereffects appeared. These results can be interpreted in the manner of previous studies. When starting position was not visible, movement was initiated in a feedforward manner with specification of the target position that also served as calibration signal and comparison of this signal with the achieved limb position prompted realignment in the proprioceptor encoder of the guided hand–head system (proprioceptive shift). Occasional reversals in the direction of linkage before the limb became visible from visual eye-to-hand guidance to proprioceptive hand-to-eye guidance produced the smaller amount of realignment in the eye–head system (visual shift).

Because of the 11.4 deg optical displacement, the initial command produced substantial error that was reduced, even on the first trial, by feedback control utilizing the visible difference between limb and target once the moving limb came into view. Subsequent improvement in exposure performance occurred by such feedback control and also because of developing realignment. However, feedback control alone is not sufficient to quickly improve performance. Moreover, realignment is slow to develop. To quickly improve performance, subjects adopted a strategy of initiating movement under feedforward control to the side of the target by the amount of error on the previous trial (knowledge-of-results compensation). Persistence of this side-pointing strategy

---

[6]This statement may not be strictly true if exteroceptors of the limb are provided with an extended tactile field or if the direction of guidance is proprioceptive (hand-to-eye), rather than visual (see chapter 6 for a more extended discussion).

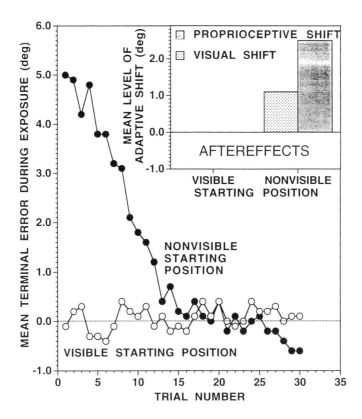

FIG. 9.5.   Feedforward control and realignment. Terminal error in pointing at a visible target during prism exposure as a function of exposure trial number for groups where the starting position for the limb was visible (feedback control) or nonvisible (feedforward and feedback control). Visual shift and proprioceptive shift aftereffects of the two groups are shown in the column graph insert. From "Contributions of Motor Control and Spatial Alignment to Prism Adaptation," by G. M.Redding and B. Wallace. In B. G. Bardy, R. J. Bootsma, and Y. Guiard (Eds.), *Studies in Perception and Action III* (p. 279), 1995, Hillsdale, NJ: Lawrence Erlbaum Associates. Copyright 1995 by Lawrence Erlbaum Associates. Adapted with permission.

after substantial realignment had developed was responsible for the overcompensation that appeared in the last few trials. Such indirect coordinative linkage also disables misalignment detection (chapters 5 and 6), and is responsible, in part, for the limited amount of realignment that occurred (chapter 7).

For the visible starting position group, exposure performance was accurate from the very first trial, but there were no realignment aftereffects. These results are consistent with the following interpretation: When both starting and target positions were visible, movement was entirely under feedback control. The visible difference between limb and target was used to zero in on the target. Because relative position of limb and target is unaffected by the optical displacement, such feedback control produced highly accurate performance.

However, under these conditions, a calibration signal to the proprioceptor encoder for the hand–head system was not necessary. No initiating target position was available for comparison with the achieved limb position and misalignment was not detected. Without a discordance signal, realignment of the proprioceptor in the hand–head system (proprioceptive shift) did not occur. Moreover, the continuously visible difference in position between limb and target (error) made it unnecessary to perform a source of error analysis and visual eye-to-hand guidance was maintained throughout the movement without any reversal in coordinative linkage. There was no hand-to-eye proprioceptive guidance that might have produced realignment in the eye–head system (visual shift).

Simultaneously visible starting and target positions is a common practice in motor control research. The present results suggest that this procedure disables adaptive alignment mechanisms. Indeed, this may be one way to isolate the contribution of strategic control to prism adaptation. However, these results also underscore the need to obtain aftereffect measures, as well as exposure performance measures, in studies of adaptive motor control employing the prism adaptation procedure.

Kinematic studies of performance during prism exposure have found the kind of trajectory correction with slow movements expected from feedback-based, error-corrective commands based on difference coding (Jakobson & Goodale, 1989). Studies of this kind also found the kind of increase in latency between end of eye saccade and onset of rapid limb movement (Rossetti et al., 1993) and change in direction of initial limb trajectory (Rossetti & Koga, 1994) expected from offline reprogramming of a position code basis for feedforward control (i.e., side-pointing).

However, without aftereffect measures we cannot know what, if any, spatial realignment occurred. Indeed, realignment aftereffects were unlikely in Jakobson and Goodale's study because starting position and target position seem to have been simultaneously visible. Realignment aftereffects should also have been small or nonexistent in Rossetti et al.'s studies, because of the rapid limb movement required and because the apparent coordination strategy was such as to disable misalignment detection. Only by comparing aftereffects and exposure performance measures are we likely to understand the relative contributions of spatial alignment and strategic control to adaptive perceptual–motor behavior.

The results of the experiments summarized here also emphasize the strategic nature of movement control codes. It seems that, depending on the task configuration, either position or difference codes or some strategic combination may be used. The view from prism adaptation research suggests a more task-dependent approach for determining the nature of movement codes.[7]

REALIGNMENT

Figure 9.6 summarizes how we think of adaptive eye–hand coordination. Representation of adaptive alignment has been attenuated in this illustration in favor of

---

[7]Abrams (1994) appeared to reach a similar conclusion.

greater elaboration of strategic control. In particular, sensory and motor encoding functions have been combined (cf. Figs. 6.1, 6.3, and 7.2) to show a single transformational operator in each subsystem (**F** and **G**), which transforms spatial coordinates in visual–motor (**VM**) space and proprioceptive–motor (**PM**) space into coordinates in noetic (**N**) space. This abbreviated representation is adequate for most instances of intersystem discordance.

Misalignment detection is illustrated in the lower left insert of Fig. 9.6 as comparison of the calibration signal received from the remote, guiding subsystem with the corresponding local spatial position. Locally detected spatial discordance activates parametric realignment of transformational operators (**G** or **F**) in the guided subsystem. The upper left insert of Fig. 9.6 illustrates the several strategic coordinative linkages possible involving eye–head and hand–head subsystems.

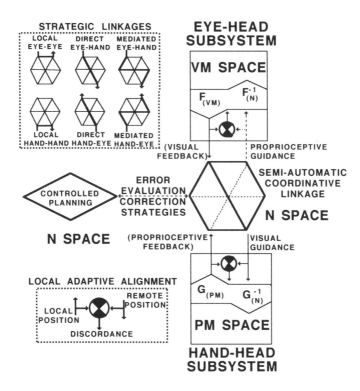

FIG. 9.6. Adaptive eye–hand coordination. Sensory and motor encoding functions have been combined to show a single transformational operator (**F** and **G**) in each subsystem that transforms spatial coordinates in visual–motor (**VM**) space and proprioceptive–motor (**PM**) space into coordinates in noetic (**N**) space. Discordance detection is illustrated in the lower left insert as comparison of the feedforward calibration signal received from the remote, guiding subsystem with the corresponding local spatial position. The insert on the upper left illustrates the several strategic coordinative linkages possible between eye–head and hand–head subsystems. Higher level strategic control includes both controlled and automatic processes for reducing performance error.

High-level strategic control includes both controlled and automatic processes for reducing performance error. Controlled planning includes the capacity for cognitively mediated linkage of eye–head and hand–head systems (e.g., side-pointing), where a position signal derived from one system is intercepted and replaced by coordinates deliberately tailored so that the responding system can achieve the target. Response coordinates are *not* target coordinates. Although such mediated linkage can reduce performance error, it is slow and capacity-limited such that it cannot operate with very high pointing rates or under secondary cognitive load.

Moreover, when the source of error is spatial misalignment, mediated linkage cannot produce realignment because there is no basis for discordance. The responding system achieves a remotely commanded position that is the same as the calibration signal used to locally interpret afference from the responding system. Mediated coordination enables rapid error reduction, but these error-reduction strategies may become nonadaptive if they persist after realignment develops.

Direct coordinative linkage is only semiautomatic because such linkage may be modulated by strategies designed to identify the source of error and monitor feedback to reduce error. Even with visual guidance tasks, coordinative linkage may be momentarily reversed to proprioceptive guidance. Such reversal permits error evaluation by visual comparison of expected and achieved limb positions and indicates appropriate reencoding or reexecution. Error-correction strategies are available for both visual guidance (e.g., zeroing out) and proprioceptive guidance (e.g., successive approximations). These strategies modify behavior in or between movements to reduce performance error.

Most importantly, when the source of error is misalignment, error correction activates local realignment in the guided system because the position required to reduce error is spatially discordant with the expected target position specified by the feedforward calibration signal. Direct coordinative linkage improves eye–hand coordination by activating realignment of subsystems as well as feedback error correction, but the latter process is typically more rapid, accounting for the larger portion of adaptive behavior.

SUMMARY

Adaptive eye–hand coordination during prism exposure reflects the joint contributions of strategic control and adaptive alignment processes. Strategic control is an immediate, but short-term solution to the performance problem posed by prismatic distortion. Whereas adaptive alignment is slower to develop, it is the long-term solution to the problem of spatial misalignment of eye–head and hand–head sensorimotor systems.

However, spatial realignment is hierarchically subordinate to strategic control and is indirectly affected by particular coordination strategies evoked by the prism exposure task. Visual feedback timing determines the direction of coordinative linkage between the misaligned systems and consequently the locus of realignment. Movement time determines the duration of coordinative linkages and therefore the amount of realignment. Cognitive load can diminish exposure performance by limiting more controlled aspects of coordination strategies. However, there may still be sufficient automatic linkage of misaligned systems to enable automatic realignment.

The contribution of strategic control to adaptive performance develops rapidly, showing complete compensation for the prismatically induced error. But persistence of such strategies in the face of more slowly developing realignment produces overcompensation. Feedforward initiation of movement with a position code is a necessary condition for realignment. Feedback control employing difference codes is, by itself, insufficient to produce realignment. Only research strategies that obtain measures of both aftereffects and exposure performance can identify the relative contributions of spatial realignment and strategic control to adaptive eye–hand coordination.

Chapter 10

IMPLICATIONS

Research in adaptive perceptual–motor performance has been characterized by insular treatments of adaptive alignment (e.g., prism adaptation) and strategic coordination (e.g., motor control). The present proposal reflects a liberal urge that is mutually heuristic, broadening in scope, and integrative in aim. Nevertheless, we believe that alignment and coordination represent distinctly separable problems (Redding & Wallace, 1993). A complete understanding of how the various, uniquely dimensional spatial representations are aligned is not likely to simply fall out from studies of normally aligned systems.

Spatial alignment should be addressed directly, and the study of adaptability to experimental misalignment (prism adaptation) is a primary means of focusing attention on this important question. On the other hand, the total adaptive response to misalignment surely involves contributions from postural adjustment and strategic control as well as realignment (Redding & Wallace, 1988c). An understanding of how these adaptive components combine will increase our knowledge of each component. We offer the present proposal as a framework in which such understanding may develop.

In this final chapter, we summarize what we believe to be the most important theoretical distinctions suggested by our analysis of prism adaptation: multiple adaptive processes, basic sensorimotor systems, and different kinds of learning. We suggest how the prism adaptation paradigm can be brought to bear on each of these theoretical issues and make some specific suggestions for further research. We conclude with a brief summary of our theoretical framework for adaptive perceptual–motor performance.

ADAPTIVE PROCESSES

Prism adaptation is not a single process. The most general distinction that has emerged from the present analysis of prism adaptation is the various, distinct adaptive processes that contribute to perceptual–motor performance. The principal categories of adaptive processes we suggested are strategic control (chapter 5), adaptive alignment (chapter 6), and postural adjustment (chapter 7).

The principle implication of these distinctions is that theory construction must allocate different aspects of adaptive performance to different processes and a complete theory must include accounts of how the various processes combine, not always in a cooperative manner, to produce adaptive performance (Redding & Wallace, 1993). Research may be focused analytically on the role of a particular process, but must include procedures that control for contributions from other processes. We have suggested several such methods.

Aftereffects can provide relatively pure measures of adaptive alignment (chapter 4) and these contributions may be subtracted from exposure performance measures to obtain an estimate of strategic control contributions (chapter 9). Of course, this requires that both aftereffects and direct effects be assessed.

However, higher level strategies deployed during prism exposure may transfer to aftereffect tests (Redding & Wallace, 1978; Welch et al., 1974). Because the conditions of similarity between exposure tasks and aftereffect tests that mediate transfer are not completely understood, component measures of realignment must be obtained for comparison with total alignment measures to enable the additivity test (chapter 4; see also chapters 8 and 9). Patterns of exposure performance and aftereffects can be predicted for different combinations of exposure task parameters (chapter 9).

For example, the observation that aftereffects do not appear when the limb can be seen from movement initiation to localization for target positions (chapter 9; Redding & Wallace, 1995, 1996a) supports the present assumptions of different control signals for feedback and feedforward control (chapters 1 and 5) and the 3-D structure of intrinsic spatial representation (chapter 2). Feedforward movement plans may be cast intrinsically in terms of the position codes necessary to detect misalignment (chapter 6), whereas feedback control may require additional computation of difference codes.

Further tests of this hypothesis could be accomplished by comparing kinematic features of pointing movements performed under exposure conditions defined by factorial combinations of visible or nonvisible starting position and prismatic displacement or no displacement (Jakobson & Goodale, 1989; Rossetti et al., 1993; see also chapter 9). No kinematic differences are expected between displacement and no displacement when the starting position is visible. Neither are realignment aftereffects expected for these conditions.

On the other hand, when the limb starting position is not visible, realignment aftereffects are expected and the kinematic record should include evidence (relative to no displacement) of feedback control (e.g., lengthening of the deceleration phase) and feedforward side-pointing utilizing knowledge of results (e.g., increased reaction time). However, these differences in aftereffects and kinematics are likely to disappear when movement time is short (less than about 200 ms), because online feedback control may be replaced by offline resetting of feedforward control in knowledge-of-results compensation (chapters 5 and 9) and because response rates of adaptive encoders may be exceeded (chapters 7 and 9).

The possibility of postural adjustment (Ebenholtz, 1974, 1976) is unavoidable in the prism adaptation paradigm (chapter 7), but control conditions that establish symmetric exercise for selected sensorimotor systems (but consequent asymmetric exercise in other systems) can be included to assess their contribution (chapter 8; see also Redding & Wallace, 1988c). For example, orthogonal manipulation of the locus of asymmetric exercise in either the eye–head or hand–head system and visual or proprioceptive guidance by early or late visual feedback (chapter 9) can be expected to produce additive contributions to aftereffect measures of postural adjustment and realignment.

Cognitive load manipulations directly affect the more controlled (attentional) aspects of strategic control (chapters 1 and 4; Redding et al., 1985), but converging operations must be included to identify particular controlled and automatic components of a coordination task (chapters 8 and 9; Redding et al., 1992). Moreover, because realignment processes are hierarchically subordinate to strategic control, aftereffect measures of realignment must be obtained to assess the indirect effects of cognitive load on adaptive spatial mapping mechanisms (chapters 8 and 9). Without such information about the contribution of realignment, exposure performance cannot be completely understood.

The intersensory-bias paradigm (chapter 7; Welch & Warren, 1980) offers a largely unexplored opportunity for identifying parameters of strategic control that may then be used to predict realignment aftereffects. Ecological bias in coordinative linkage reflected by dominance relationships among sensorimotor systems should determine the locus and relative magnitude of realignment obtained with the prism adaptation paradigm.

SENSORIMOTOR SYSTEMS

Perhaps most controversial is the particular sensorimotor systems suggested by the present analysis of prism adaptation research. There is considerable logical, neurological, and behavioral evidence for the eye–head as a distinct sensorimotor system (chapter 1), but the evidential bases for other systems like the hand–head is much less clear. Complicating such identification is the likelihood that sensorimotor systems can be differently organized into task-specific, superordinate, functional systems.

Indeed, it seems likely to us that the hand–head is a functional organization, composed of several basic sensorimotor systems, perhaps structurally defined by the several joints (chapters 2 and 4). The idea of a basic sensorimotor system (chapters 1 and 6) that is capable of autonomous orienting behavior offers a means of identifying the fundamental organizational units of the perceptual–motor system.

Obtaining aftereffect measures in the prism adaptation paradigm is one method for identifying basic sensorimotor systems. Only such systems can show localized realignment that combine additively to produce the total realignment in a functionally organized system. Aftereffects at different points in a basic system will have the same magnitude, and any local test will show the same magnitude as an overall test of the coordination loop.

For example, an invariant pattern of additivity for local aftereffects in the hand–head system (e.g., hand–wrist, forearm–elbow, upperarm–shoulder, shoulder–head) over different coordination tasks would constitute strong evidence for the basic nature of these sensorimotor systems. However, if the hand–head is itself a basic system, local tests will show the same aftereffect and the same as the hand–head aftereffect. The sum of local aftereffects will exceed the total aftereffect. Such behavioral data would facilitate identification of the underlying neural circuitry. Further application of this methodology should enable identification of basic sensorimotor units in the auditory and locomotion systems (chapters 6 and 8).

The prism adaptation paradigm also provides a means of investigating the internal organization of basic sensorimotor systems. For example, investigations of the distinction between exteroceptor and proprioceptive realignment (chapters 6 and 7) could be undertaken by orthogonal exposure manipulations of the extension of exteroceptor fields and the occurrence or nonoccurrence of corrective movements. Size of the exteroceptor field might be manipulated by a lighted versus reduced visual field or by comparing an extended tactile field like the palm of the hand with a reduced field like the fingertip. Instructions or cognitive load might be sufficient to prevent corrective movements.

Adaptive encoders for exteroceptors and proprioceptors are likely to have different response characteristics. An extended exteroceptor field without corrective movement should produce exteroceptor realignment that is parametrically different from proprioceptor realignment produced by an extended exteroceptor field with corrective movement. A reduced exteroceptor field with corrective movement should produce proprioceptor realignment, but the absence of corrective movement with a reduced exteroceptor field may not produce realignment of either kind. Moreover, the distinguishing parametric characteristics of exteroceptor and proprioceptor realignment are likely to be different for different sensorimotor systems. Of course, aftereffect tests of realignment must be specific to the particular sensorimotor system that is the target of the manipulation (e.g., visual or proprioceptive shift tests).

LEARNING

Perhaps the most fundamental distinction suggested by our analysis of prism adaptation is between the two kinds of learning: associative rule learning and nonassociative parametric learning (chapters 2, 3, 5, and 6; Bedford, 1993b). While we believe that the evidence is strong for distinct strategic control and spatial alignment processes (chapters 8 and 9), the evidence that different kinds of learning are involved is more limited.

The principal source of such evidence is research showing different generalization functions for different learning tasks (chapters 2 and 3; Bedford, 1989, 1993a). Of course, the point of these studies is to determine the kinds of mapping rules (transformations) that are innately given and for which parameters may be learned (i.e. showing complete generalization). These rules can then be contrasted with mapping rules that must themselves be learned (i.e., showing graded generalization).

Still, from the present perspective, such studies have the difficulty that they confound unknown task differences with differences in learning (mapping rules).

Because we believe that both kinds of learning are evoked by the usual prism adaptation task (chapters 4 and 9), a more convincing methodology would test for differences in generalization among the adaptive components of performance during prism exposure, identifying different kinds of learning for the same training task.

The distinction between associative and nonassociative learning could be tested by comparing generalization in training and in aftereffect tests. The present proposal predicts that feedforward strategies like side-pointing deployed during training are associative in nature and should show typical generalization gradients. Realignment measured by aftereffects are nonassociative and should show complete generalization.

For example, after a period of single-point training in eye–hand coordination (e.g., Bedford, 1989), a transfer task that is indistinguishable from training except that a different point is tested should show a generalization gradient. In contrast, a total shift aftereffect test distinguishable by complete removal of training context (e.g., the prism-bearing goggles) should show more complete generalization for a test point that is different from either training or transfer points. The generalization gradient for the transfer test should become even more apparent if the contribution of realignment measured by the aftereffect test is subtracted (chapter 9). Converging evidence of realignment as well as its locus could be provided by the addition of the traditional visual and proprioceptive shift tests, thereby enabling the additivity test (chapter 4).

A further test could be conducted by acquiring visual, proprioceptive, and total shift measures during each no-displacement phase in contextually distinctive, no-displacement–displacement training cycles of an eye–hand coordination task (chapter 5; Bingham et al., 1991; Bridgeman et al., 1992). As initial error for each displacement phase decreases, indicating associative learning, aftereffect measures should decrease. Deployment of a context-specific side-pointing strategy disables misalignment detection (chapters 6 and 9). Moreover, the total shift that remains may exceed the sum of visual and proprioceptive shift early in training, indicating transfer of associative learning of the training task to the similar total shift aftereffect test (chapters 4 and 9) before contextual discrimination of training phases is complete.

SUMMARY

Postural adjustment, spatial alignment, and strategic control are levels of a hierarchy of processes that serve adaptive perceptual–motor performance. At the lowest, most peripheral level, postural adjustments are short-latency adaptive responses to changes in environmental load on muscle systems. Such load compensation may be activated by changes in patterned innervation of muscle systems occasioned by the asymmetric exercise required for coordinated behavior under conditions of spatial misalignment.

At the highest, most central level, strategic control is the task-oriented conjoining of sensorimotor subsystems to achieve common action. Such feedback-sensitive processes may be rapidly deployed to reduce performance error caused by spatial misalignment.

At the intermediate level, realignment is the long-latency response to spatial misalignment of local transformational operators that normally serve to translate among unique sensorimotor spaces. Misalignment is detected by local comparison, in a guided sensorimotor subsystem, between the position expected on the basis of a remote signal from the guiding subsystem and the corresponding local position required of the guided subsystem. Such feedforward discordance detection and realignment is critically dependent on direct coordinative linkages that pass corresponding positional information between subsystems. Experimental misalignment recruits an array of adaptive processes and provides an opportunity to investigate the complexity of adaptive perceptual–motor performance.

REFERENCES

Abbs, J. H., Gracco, V. L., & Cole, K. J. (1984). Control of multimovement coordination: Sensorimotor mechanisms in speech motor programming. *Journal of Motor Behavior, 16,* 195–231.

Abbs, J. H., & Winstein, C. J. (1990). Functional contributions of rapid and automatic sensory-based adjustments to motor output. In M. Jeannerod (Ed.), *Attention and performance XII: Motor representation and control* (pp. 627–652). Hillsdale, NJ: Lawrence Erlbaum Associates.

Abend, W. M., Bizzi, E., & Morasso, P. (1982). Human arm trajectory formation. *Brain, 105,* 331–348.

Abrams, R. A. (1994). Eye–hand coordination: Spatial localization after saccadic and pursuit eye movements. *Journal of Motor Behavior, 26,* 215–224.

Adams, J. A. (1971). A closed-loop theory of motor behavior. *Journal of Motor Behavior, 3,* 111–149.

Adams, J. A. (1991). The changing face of motor learning. In R. B. Wilberg (Ed.), *The learning, memory, and perception of perceptual-motor skills* (pp. 3–14). Amsterdam: North-Holland. (Original work published 1990).

Anderson, J. R. (1983). *The architecture of cognition.* Cambridge, MA: Harvard University Press.

Anderson, J. R. (1987). Skill acquisition: Compilation of weak-method problem solutions. *Psychological Review, 94,* 192–210.

Annett, J., Golby, C. W., & Kay, H. (1958). The measurements of elements in an assembly task: The information output of the human motor system. *Quarterly Journal of Experimental Psychology, 10,* 1–11.

Arbib, M. A. (1972). *The metaphorical brain.* New York: Wiley.

Arbib, M. A. (1981). Perceptual structures and distributed motor control. In V. B. Brooks (Ed.), *Handbook of physiology: Sec. 1, The nervous system; Vol. II, Motor control, Pt. 2* (pp. 1449–1480). Bethesda, MD: American Physiological Society.

Auerbach, C., & Sperling, P. (1974). A common auditory–visual space: Evidence for its reality. *Perception and Psychophysics, 16,* 129–135.

Baily, J. S. (1972). Adaptation to prisms: Do proprioceptive changes mediate adapted behavior with ballistic arm movements? *Quarterly Journal of Experimental Psychology, 24,* 8–20.

Barr, C. C., Schultheis, L. W., & Robinson, D. A. (1976). Voluntary, non-visual control of the human vestibulo-ocular reflex. *Acta Otolaryngology, 81,* 365–375.

Basmajian, J. V., & De Luca, C. J. (1985). *Muscles alive: Their functions revealed by electromyography* (5th ed.). Baltimore, MD: Williams & Wilkins.

Beaubaton, D., & Hay, L. (1986). Contribution of visual information to feedforward and feedback processes in rapid pointing movements. *Human Movement Science, 5,* 19–34.

Beckett, P. A. (1980). Development of the third component in prism adaptation: Effect of active and passive movement. *Journal of Experimental Psychology: Human Perception and Performance, 6,* 433–444.

Beckett, P. A., Melamed, L. E., & Halay, M. (1975, May). *Prism awareness, exposure duration, and the linear model in prism adaptation.* Paper presented at meeting of the Midwestern Psychological Association, Chicago, IL.

Bedford, F. (1989). Constraints on learning new mapping between perceptual dimensions. *Journal of Experimental Psychology: Human Perception and Performance, 15,* 232–248.

Bedford, F. (1993a). Perceptual and cognitive spatial learning. *Journal of Experimental Psychology: Human Perception and Performance, 19,* 517–530.

Bedford, F. (1993b). Perceptual learning. In D. Medin (Ed.), *Psychology of learning and motivation; Advances in research and theory* (Vol. 30, pp. 1–60). New York: Academic Press.

Bedford, F. (1994). A pair of paradoxes and the perceptual pairing process. *Cahiers de Psychologie/Current Psychology of Cognition, 13,* 60–68.

Bedford, F., & Reinke, K. S. (1993). The McCollough Effect: Dissociating retinal from spatial coordinations. *Perception and Psychophysics, 54,* 515–526.

Beggs, W. D. A., & Howarth, C. I. (1972). The movement of the hand toward a target. *Quarterly Journal of Experimental Psychology, 24,* 448–453.

Berkenblit, M. B., Feldman, A. G., & Fucson, O. I. (1986). Adaptability of innate motor patterns and motor control. *Behavioral and Brain Sciences, 9,* 585–638.

Bernstein, N. (1967). *The coordination and regulation of movement.* New York: Pergamon.

Biederman, I. (1985). Human image understanding: Recent research and theory. *Computer Vision, Graphics, and Image Processing, 32,* 29–73.

Biederman, I. (1987). Recognition-by-components: A theory of human image understanding. *Psychological Review, 94,* 115–147.

Biederman, I. (1990). Higher-level vision. In D. N. Osherson, S. M. Kosslyn, & J. M. Hollerbach (Eds.), *An invitation to cognitive science: Vol. 2, Visual cognition and action* (pp. 41–72). Cambridge, MA: MIT Press.

Biguer, B., Jeannerod, M., & Prablanc, C. (1982). The coordination of eye, head, and arm movements during reaching at a single target. *Experimental Brain Research, 46,* 301–304.

Biguer, B., Jeannerod, M., & Prablanc, C. (1985). The role of position of gaze in movement accuracy. In M. I. Posner & O. S. Marin (Eds.), *Attention and performance XI: Mechanisms of attention* (pp. 407–424). Hillsdale, NJ: Lawrence Erlbaum Associates.

Bingham, G. P., Muchisky, M., & Romack, J. L. (1991, November). *"Adaptation" to displacement prisms is skill acquisition.* Paper presented at the 32nd Annual Meeting of the Psychonomic Society, San Francisco, CA.

Bizzi, E. (1980). Central and peripheral mechanisms in motor control. In G. E. Stelmach & J. Requin (Eds.), *Tutorials in motor behavior* (pp. 131–143). New York: North-Holland.

Bonnet, M., Requin, J., & Stelmach, G. E. (1982). Specification of direction and extent in motor programming. *Bulletin of the Psychonomic Society, 19,* 31–34.

Bridgeman, B., Anand, S., Browman, K. E., & Welch, R. B. (1992, November). *Necessary conditions for speeded visuomotor adaptation.* Paper presented at the 33rd Annual Meeting of the Psychonomic Society, St. Louis, MO.

Buchanan, T. S., Almdale, D. P. J., Lewis, J. L., & Rymer, W. Z. (1986). Characteristics of synergic relations during isometric contractions of human elbow muscles. *Journal of Neurophysiology, 56,* 1225–1241.

Bullock, D., & Grossberg, S. (1988). Neural dynamics of planned arm movements: Emergent invariants and speed–accuracy properties during trajectory formation. *Psychological Review, 95,* 49–90.

Bullock, D., & Grossberg, S. (1989). VITE and FLETE: Neural modules for trajectory formation and postural control. In W. A. Hershberger (Ed.), *Volitional action* (pp. 253–297). Amsterdam: North-Holland-Elsevier.

Bullock, D., Grossberg, S., & Guenther, F. H. (1993). A self-organizing neural model of motor equivalent reaching and tool use by a multijoint arm. *Journal of Cognitive Neuroscience, 5,* 408–435.

Canon, L. K. (1970). Intermodality inconsistency of input and directed attention as determinants of the nature of adaptation. *Journal of Experimental Psychology, 84,* 141–147.

Canon, L. K. (1971). Directed attention and maladaptive "adaptation" to displacement of the visual field. *Journal of Experimental Psychology, 88,* 403–408.

Carlton, L. G. (1992). Visual processing time and the control of movement. In L. Proteau & D. Elliott (Eds.), *Vision and motor control* (pp. 3–31). Amsterdam: Elsevier Science Publishers.

Churchland, P. S. (1986). *Neurophilosophy: Toward a unified science of the mind/brain.* Cambridge, MA: MIT Press.

Cohen, H. B. (1966). Some critical issues in prism adaptation. *American Journal of Psychology, 79,* 285–290.

Cohen, M. M. (1967). Continuous versus terminal visual feedback in prism aftereffects. *Perceptual and Motor Skills, 24,* 1295–1302.

Coren, S. (1966). Adaptation to prismatic displacement as a function of the amount of available information. *Psychonomic Science, 4,* 407–408.

Craske, B. (1967). Adaptation to prisms: Change in internally registered eye-position. *British Journal of Psychology, 58,* 329–335.

Craske, B. (1975). A current view of the processes and mechanisms of prism adaptation. *Les Colloques de l'Institut National de la Santé et de la Recherche Médicale, 43,* 125–138.

Craske, B. (1977). Perception of impossible limb positions induced by tendon vibration. *Science, 196,* 71–73.

Craske, B. (1981). Programmed aftereffects following simple patterned movements of the eyes and limbs. In J. Long & A. Baddeley (Eds.), *Attention and performance IX* (pp. 473–485). Hillsdale, NJ: Lawrence Erlbaum Associates.

Craske, B., & Crawshaw, M. (1974). Adaptive changes of opposite sign in the oculomotor systems of the two eyes. *Quarterly Journal of Experimental Psychology, 26,* 106–113.

Craske, B., & Crawshaw, M. (1978). Spatial discordance is a sufficient condition for oculomotor adaptation to prisms: Eye muscle potentiation need not be a factor. *Perception and Psychophysics, 23,* 75–79.

Craske, B., Crawshaw, M., & Heron, P. (1975). Disturbance of the oculomotor system due to lateral fixation. *Quarterly Journal of Experimental Psychology, 27,* 459–465.

Craske, B., & Gregg, S. J. (1966). Prism after-effects: Identical results for visual targets and unexposed limb. *Nature, 212,* 104–105.

Crawshaw, M., & Craske, B. (1974). No retinal component in prism adaptation. *Acta Psychologica, 38,* 421–423.

Crossman, E. R. F. W., & Goodeve, P. J. (1963/1983). Feedback control of hand-movement and Fitts' Law. Paper presented at the meeting of the Experimental Psychology Society, Oxford, July 1963. *Quarterly Journal of Experimental Psychology, 1983, 35A,* 251–278.

Cruse, H. (1986). Constraints for joint angle control of the human arm. *Biological Cybernetics, 54,* 125–132.

Cunningham, H. A. (1989). Aiming error under transformed spatial mappings suggests a structure for visual-motor maps. *Journal of Experimental Psychology: Human Perception and Performance, 15,* 493–506.

Cutting, J. E. (1986). *Perception with an eye for motion.* Cambridge, MA: MIT Press.

Dewar, R. (1970). Adaptation to displaced vision: Amount of optical displacement and practice. *Perception and Psychophysics, 8,* 313–316.

Dewar, R. (1971). Adaptation to displaced vision: Variations on the "prismatic shaping" technique. *Perception and Psychophysics, 9,* 155–157.

Dodwell, P. C. (1970). *Visual pattern recognition.* New York: Holt, Rinehart & Winston.

Ebenholtz, S. M. (1966). Adaptation to a rotated visual field as a function of degree of optical tilt and exposure time. *Journal of Experimental Psychology, 72,* 629–634.

Ebenholtz, S. M. (1973). Optimal input rates for tilt adaptation. *American Journal of Psychology, 86,* 193–200.

Ebenholtz, S. M. (1974). The possible role of eye-muscle potentiation in several forms of prism adaptation. *Perception, 3,* 477–485.

Ebenholtz, S. M. (1976). Additivity of aftereffects of maintained head and eye rotations: An alternative to recalibration. *Perception and Psychophysics, 19,* 113–116.

Ebenholtz, S. M., & Callan, J. W. (1980). Tilt adaptation as a feedback control process. *Journal of Experimental Psychology: Human Perception and Performance, 6,* 413–432.

Ebenholtz, S. M., & Fisher, S. K. (1982). Distance adaptation depends upon plasticity in the oculomotor control system. *Perception and Psychophysics, 31,* 551–560.

Ebenholtz, S. M., & Mayer, D. (1968). Rate of adaptation under constant and varied optical tilt. *Perceptual and Motor Skill, 26,* 507–509.

Ebenholtz, S. M., & Redding, G. M. (1970). Temporal characteristics of a comparator in adaptation to optical tilt. *Perception and Psychophysics, 7,* 365–366.

Ebenholtz, S. M., & Wolfson, D. M. (1975). Perceptual aftereffects of sustained convergence. *Perception and Psychophysics, 17,* 485–491.

Efstathiou, E. (1969). Effects of exposure time and magnitude of prism transform on eye–hand coordination. *Journal of Experimental Psychology, 81,* 235–240.

Efstathiou, E., Bauer, J., Greene, M., & Held, R. (1967). Altered reaching following adaptation to optical displacement. *Journal of Experimental Psychology, 73,* 113–120.

Elliott, D. (1988). The influence of visual target and limb information on manual aiming. *Canadian Journal of Psychology, 42,* 57–68.

Elliott, D. (1992). Intermittent versus continuous control of manual aiming movements. In L. Proteau & D. Elliott (Eds.), *Vision and motor control* (pp. 33–48). Amsterdam: North-Holland.

Elliott, D., Carson, R. G., Goodman, D., & Chua, R. (1991). Discrete vs. continuous control of manual aiming. *Human Movement Science, 10,* 393–418.

Ells, J. G. (1973). Analysis of temporal and attentional aspects of movement control. *Journal of Experimental Psychology, 99,* 10–21.

Epstein, W. (1967). *Varieties of perceptual learning.* New York: McGraw Hill.

Epstein, W. (1975). Recalibration by pairing: A process of perceptual learning. *Perception, 4,* 59–72.

Epstein, W., & Morgan, C. L. (1970). Adaptation to uniocular image magnification: Modification of the disparity–depth relationship. *American Journal of Psychology, 83,* 322–329.

Epstein, W., & Morgan-Paap, C. L. (1974). The effect of level of depth processing and degree of informational discrepancy on adaptation to uniocular image magnification. *Journal of Experimental Psychology, 102,* 585–594.

Epstein, W., & Park, J. N. (1963). Shape constancy: Functional relationships and theoretical formulations. *Psychological Bulletin, 60,* 265–288.

Epstein, W., Park, J., & Casey, A. (1961). The current status of the size–distance hypotheses. *Psychological Bulletin, 38,* 491–514.

Ezure, K., &´Graf, W. (1984a). A quantitative analysis of the spatial organization of the vestibulo-ocular reflexes in lateral- and frontal-eyed animals: I. Orientation of semicircular canals and extraocular muscles. *Neuroscience, 12,* 85–93.

Ezure, K., & Graf, W. (1984b). A quantitative analysis of spatial organization of the vestibulo-ocular reflexes in lateral- and frontal-eyed animals: II. Neuronal networks underlying vestibulo-oculomotor coordination. *Neuroscience, 12,* 95–109.

Farah, M. J. (1989). Mechanisms of imagery–perception interaction. *Journal of Experimental Psychology: Human Perception and Performance, 15,* 203–211.

Favilla, M., Hening, W., & Ghez, C. (1989). Trajectory control in targeted force impulses. VI. Independent separation of response amplitude and direction. *Experimental Brain Research, 75,* 280–294.

Feldman, A. G. (1986). Once more on the equilibrium-point hypothesis (λ model) for motor control. *Journal of Motor Behavior, 18,* 17–54.

Feltz, D. L., & Landers, D. M. (1983). The effects of mental practice on motor skill learning and performance: A meta-analysis. *Journal of Sport Psychology, 5,* 25–57.

Festinger, L., Burnham, C. A., Ono, H., & Bamber, D. (1967). Efference and the conscious experience of perception. *Journal of Experimental Psychology Monographs, 74,* 4, Pt. 2.

Fisher, G. H. (1962a). *Intersensory localization.* Unpublished doctoral thesis, University of Hull, England.

Fisher, G. H. (1962b). Resolution of spatial conflict. *Bulletin of the British Psychological Society, 46,* 3A.

Fisher, G. H. (1968). *The frameworks for perceptual localization.* Report of Ministry of Defence research project (No. 70/GEN/9617). University of Newcastle upon Tyne, England.

Fishkin, S. M. (1969). Passive vs. active exposure and other variables related to the occurrence of hand adaptation to lateral displacement. *Perceptual and Motor Skills, 29,* 291–297.

Fitch, H. L., Tuller, B., & Turvey, M. T. (1982). The Bernstein perspective: III. Tuning of coordinative structures with special reference to perception. In J. A. S. Kelso (Ed.), *Human motor behavior* (pp. 271–281). Hillsdale, NJ: Lawrence Erlbaum Associates.

Fitts, P. M. (1954). The information capacity of the human motor system in controlling the amplitude of movement. *Journal of Experimental Psychology, 47,* 381–391.

Fitts, P. M. (1964). Perceptual–motor skills learning. In A. W. Melton (Ed.), *Categories of human learning* (pp. 243–285). New York: Academic Press.

Fitts, P. M., Bahrick, H. P., Noble, M. E., & Briggs, G. E. (1961). *Skilled performance.* New York: Wiley.

Fitts, P. M., & Peterson, J. R. (1964). Information capacity of discrete motor responses. *Journal of Experimental Psychology, 67,* 103–112.

Flanders, M., & Soechting, J. F. (1990). Parcellation of sensorimotor transformations for arm movements. *Journal of Neuroscience, 10,* 2420–2427.

Flash, T., & Hogan, N. (1985). The coordination of arm movements: An experimentally confirmed mathematical model. *Journal of Neuroscience, 5,* 1688–1703.

Fodor, J. A. (1983). *The modularity of mind.* Cambridge, MA: MIT Press.

Foley, J. E., & Maynes, F. J. (1969). Comparison of training methods in the production of prism adaptation. *Journal of Experimental Psychology, 81,* 151–155.

Fowler, C. A., & Turvey, M. T. (1978). Skill acquisition: An event approach with special reference to searching for the optimum of a function of several variables. In G. E. Stelmach (Ed.), *Information processing in motor control and learning* (pp. 1–40). New York: Academic Press.

Freedman, S. J. (1968). Perceptual compensation and learning. In S. J. Freedman (Ed.), *The neuropsychology of spatially oriented behavior* (pp. 63–76). Homewood, IL: Dorsey.

Fu, Q.-G., Suarez, J. L., & Ebner, T. J. (1993). Neuronal specification of direction and distance during reaching movements in the superior precentral premotor area and primary motor cortex in monkeys. *Journal of Neurophysiology, 70, 5,* 2097–2116.

Fuchs, A. H. (1962). The progression–regression hypothesis in perceptual-motor skill learning. *Journal of Experimental Psychology, 63,* 177–182.

Fullerton, G. S., & Cattell, J. M. (1892). *On the perception of small differences: With special reference to the extent, force, and time of movement.* Philadelphia, PA: University of Pennsylvania Press.

Gaudiano, P., & Grossberg, S. (1991). Vector associative maps: Unsupervised real-time error-based learning and control of movement trajectories. *Neural Networks, 4,* 147–183.

Gauthier, G. M., Vercher, J-L., Mussa-Ivaldi, F., & Marchetti, E. (1988). Oculo-manual tracking of visual targets: Control learning, coordination control and coordination model. *Experimental Brain Research, 73,* 127–137.

Georgopoulos, A. P. (1986). On reaching. *Annual Review of Neuroscience, 9,* 147–170.

Georgopoulos, A. P. (1990). Neurophysiology of reaching. In M. Jeannerod (Ed.), *Attention and performance XII: Motor representation and control* (pp. 227–263). Hillsdale, NJ: Lawrence Erlbaum Associates.

Georgopoulos, A. P., Kalaska, J. F., Caminiti, R., & Massey, J. T. (1982). On the relations between the direction of two-dimensional arm movements and cell discharge in primate motor cortex. *Journal of Neuroscience, 2,* 1527–1537.

Gibson, E. J. (1969). *Principles of perceptual learning and development.* New York: Appleton-Century-Crofts.

Gibson, E. J. (1984). Perceptual development from the ecological approach. In M. E. Lamb, A. L. Brown, & B. Rogoff (Eds.), *Advances in developmental psychology, Vol. 3* (pp. 243–286). Hillsdale, NJ: Lawrence Erlbaum Associates.

Gibson, J. J. (1950). *The perception of the visual world.* Boston, MA: Houghton Mifflin.

Gibson, J. J. (1966). *The senses considered as perceptual systems.* Boston, MA: Houghton Mifflin.

Gibson, J. J. (1979). *The ecological approach to visual perception.* Boston, MA: Houghton Mifflin.

Goodale, M. A., Milner, A. D., Jakobson, L. S., Carey, D. P. (1990). Kinematic analysis of limb movements in neuropsychological research: Subtle deficits and recovery of function. *Canadian Journal of Psychology, 44,* 180–195.

Goodale, M. A., Pélisson, D., & Prablanc, C. (1986). Large adjustments in visually guided reaching do not depend on vision of the hand or perception of target displacement. *Nature, 320,* 748–750.

Goodwin, G. M., McCloskey, D. I., & Matthews, P. B. C. (1972). The contribution of muscle afferents to kinesthesia shown by vibration induced illusions of movement and by the effects of paralyzing joint afferents. *Brain, 95,* 705–748.

Greene, M. E. (1967, April). *A further study of the proprioceptive change hypothesis of prism adaptation.* Paper presented at meetings of the Eastern Psychological Association, Boston, MA.

Greene, P. H. (1969). Seeking mathematical models for skilled actions. In D. Bootzin & H. C. Muffley (Eds.), *Biomechanics* (pp. 149–180). New York: Plenum.

Greene, P. H. (1972). Problems of organization of motor systems. In R. Rosen & F. M. Snell (Ed.), *Progress in theoretical biology* (Vol. 2, pp. 303–338). New York: Academic Press.

Greene, P. H. (1982). Why is it easy to control your arms? *Journal of Motor Behavior, 14,* 260–286.

Grobstein, P. (1988). Between the retinotectal projection and directed movement: Topography of a sensorimotor interface. *Brain, Behavior, and Evolution, 31,* 34–48.

Grossberg, S., & Kuperstein, M. (1989). *Neural dynamics of adaptive sensory–motor control: Expanded edition.* New York: Pergamon.

Hall, G. (1991). *Perceptual and associative learning.* Oxford: Clarendon Press.

Hamilton, C. R. (1964). *Studies of adaptation to deflection of the visual field in split-brain monkeys and man.* Unpublished doctoral dissertation, California Institute of Technology, Pasadena, CA.

Hardt, M. E., Held, R., & Steinbach, M. J. (1971). Adaptation to displaced vision: A change in central control of sensorimotor coordination. *Journal of Experimental Psychology, 89,* 229–239.

Harris, C. S. (1963). Adaptation to displaced vision: Visual, motor, or proprioceptive change? *Science, 140,* 812–813.

Harris, C. S. (1965). Perceptual adaptation to inverted, reversed, and displaced vision. *Psychological Review, 72,* 419–444.

Harvey, N. L., & Greer, K. (1980). Action: The mechanisms of motor control. In G. L. Claxton (Ed.), *Cognitive psychology: New directions* (pp. 65–111). London: Routledge and Kegan Paul.

Hasher, L., & Zacks, R. T. (1979). Automatic and effortful processes in memory. *Journal of Experimental Psychology: General, 108,* 356–388.

Hay, J. C. (1974). Motor-transformation learning. *Perception, 3,* 487–496.

Hay, J. C., Langdon, B., & Pick, H. L, Jr. (1971). Spatial parameters of eye–hand adaptation to optical distortion. *Journal of Experimental Psychology, 91,* 11–17.

Hay, J. C., & Pick, H. L., Jr. (1966a). Gaze-contingent prism adaptation: Optical and motor factors. *Journal of Experimental Psychology, 72,* 640–648.

Hay, J. C., & Pick, H. L., Jr. (1966b). Visual and proprioceptive adaptation to optical displacement of the visual stimulus. *Journal of Experimental Psychology, 71,* 150–158.

Hay, L. (1970). *Contribution à l'étude de l'organisation de l'espace postural chez l'Homme: Étude expérimentale de l'adaptation des différents segments du corps à une déviation prismatique du champ visuel* [Contribution to the study of the organization of postural space in man: Experimental study of the adaptation of different body segments to a prismatic displacement of the visual field.] *Cahiers de Psychologie, 13,* 3–24.

Hay, L., & Brouchon, M. (1972). *Analyse de la réorganisation des coordinations visuo-motrices chez l'homme* [Analysis of the reorganization of visual-motor coordination in man.] *L'Année Psychologique (Paris), 72,* 25–38.

Hebb, D. O. (1949). *The organization of behavior.* New York: Wiley.

Hein, A. (1972). Acquiring components of visually guided behavior. In A. D. Pick (Ed.), *Minnesota symposium on child psychology* (pp. 53–68). Minneapolis: University of Minnesota Press.

Hein, A., & Held, R. (1962). A neural model for labile sensorimotor coordinations. In E. E. Bernard & M. R. Kare (Ed.), *Biological prototypes and synthetic systems* (Vol. 1, pp. 71–74). New York: Plenum.

Held, R. (1961). Exposure-history as a factor in maintaining stability of perception and co-ordination. *Journal of Nervous and Mental Disease, 132,* 26–32.

Held, R. (1968). Dissociation of visual functions by deprivation and rearrangement. *Psychologische Forschung, 31,* 338–348.

Held, R. (1980). The rediscovery of adaptability in the visual system: Effects of intrinsic and extrinsic chromatic dispersion. In C. S. Harris (Ed.), *Visual coding and adaptability* (pp. 69–94). Hillsdale, NJ: Lawrence Erlbaum Associates.

Held, R., & Bossom, J. (1961). Neonatal deprivation and adult rearrangement: Complementary techniques for analyzing plastic sensory–motor coordination. *Journal of Comparative and Physiological Psychology, 54,* 33–37.

Held, R. & Freedman, S. J. (1963). Plasticity in human sensorimotor control. *Science, 142,* 455–462.

Held, R., & Gottlieb, N. (1958). Technique for studying adaptation to disarranged hand–eye coordination. *Perceptual and Motor Skills, 8,* 83–86.

Held, R., & Hein, A. (1958). Adaptation to disarranged hand–eye coordination contingent upon reafferent stimulation. *Perceptual and Motor Skills, 8,* 87–90.

Held, R., & Mikaelian, H. (1964). Motor-sensory feedback versus need in adaptation to rearrangement. *Perceptual and Motor Skills, 18,* 685–688.

Held, R., & Schlank, M. (1959). Adaptation to disarranged eye-hand coordination in the distance dimension. *American Journal of Psychology, 72,* 603–605.

Helmholtz, H. E. F. von (1962). *Treatise on physiological optics.* (J. P. C. Southall, Ed. and Trans.). New York: Dover. (Original work published in 1909)

Henry, F. M. (1968). Specificity vs. generality in learning motor skill. In R. C. Brown & G. S. Kenyon (Eds.), *Classical studies on physical activity* (pp. 331–340). Englewood Cliffs, NJ: Prentice-Hall.

Hildreth, E. C. (1984a). Computations underlying the measurement of visual motion. *Artificial Intelligence, 23,* 309–354.

Hildreth, E. C. (1984b). The computation of the velocity field. *Proceedings of the Royal Society of London B 221,* 189–354.

Hogan, N., & Flash, T. (1987). Moving gracefully: Quantitative theories of motor coordination. *Trends in the Neurosciences, 10,* 170–174.

Houk, J. C., & Rymer, W. Z. (1981). Neural control of muscle length and tension. In V. B. Brooks (Ed.), *Handbook of Physiology: Sec. 1. The nervous system; Vol. 2. Motor Control, Pt. 1* (pp. 257–323). Bethesda, MD: American Physiological Society.

Howard, I. P. (1967, November). *Response shaping to visual–motor discordance.* Paper presented at the meeting of the Psychonomic Society, Chicago, IL.

Howard, I. P. (1971a). The adaptability of the visual-motor system. In K. J. Connolly (Ed.), *Mechanisms of motor skill development* (pp. 337–352). London: Academic Press.

Howard, I. P. (1971b). Perceptual learning and adaptation. *British Medical Bulletin, 27,* 248–252.

Howard, I. P. (1982). *Human visual orientation.* New York: Wiley.

Howard, I. P., & Anstis, T. (1974). Muscular and joint-receptor components of postural persistence. *Journal of Experimental Psychology, 103,* 167–170.

Howard, I. P., Anstis, T., & Lucia, H. C. (1974). The relative lability of mobile and stationary components in a visual–motor adaptation task. *Quarterly Journal of Experimental Psychology, 26,* 293–300.

Howard, I. P., Craske, B., & Templeton, W. B. (1965). Visuo-motor adaptation to discordant exafferent stimulation. *Journal of Experimental Psychology, 70,* 189–191.

Howard, I. P., & Templeton, W. B. (1966). *Human spatial orientation.* New York: Wiley.

Jackendoff, R., & Landau, B. (1994). What is coded in parietal representations? *Behavioral and Brain Sciences* [commentary], *17,* 211–212.

Jakobson, L. S., & Goodale, M. A. (1989). Trajectories of reaches to prismatically-displaced targets: Evidence for "automatic" visuomotor recalibration. *Experimental Brain Research, 78,* 575–587.

James, W. (1890). *The principles of psychology* (Vol. 1). New York: Holt.

Jeannerod, M. (1981). Intersegmental coordination during reaching at natural visual objects. In J. Long & A. Baddeley (Eds.), *Attention and performance IX* (pp. 153–168). Hillsdale, NJ: Lawrence Erlbaum Associates.

Jeannerod, M. (1984). The timing of natural prehension movements. *Journal of Motor Behavior, 16,* 235–254.

Jeannerod, M. (1986a). The formation of finger grip during prehension: A cortically mediated visuomotor pattern. *Behavioral Brain Research, 19,* 99–116

Jeannerod, M. (1986b). Mechanisms of visuomotor coordination: A study in normal and brain-damaged subjects. *Neuropsychologia, 24,* 41–78.

Jeannerod, M. (1988). *The neural and behavioral organization of goal-directed movements.* New York: Oxford University Press.

Jeannerod, M. (1991a). The interaction of visual and proprioceptive cues in controlling reaching movements. In D. R. Humphrey & H. J. Freund (Eds.), *Motor control: Concepts and issues* (pp. 277–291). New York: Wiley.

Jeannerod, M. (1991b). A neurophysiological model for the directional coding of reaching movements. In J. Paillard (Ed.), *Brain and space* (pp. 49–69). New York: Oxford University Press.

Jeannerod, M. (1992). Coordination mechanisms in prehension movements. In G. E. Stelmach & J. Requin (Eds.), *Tutorials in motor behavior II* (pp. 265–285). Amsterdam: Elsevier Science.

Jeannerod, M. (1994). The representing brain: Neural correlates of motor intention and imagery. *Behavioral and Brain Sciences, 17,* 187–245.

Jeannerod, M., & Biguer, B. (1982). Visuomotor mechanisms in reaching within extrapersonal space. In D. J. Ingle, M. A. Goodale, & R. J. W. Mansfield (Eds.), *Analysis of visual behavior* (pp. 387–409). Cambridge, MA: MIT Press.

Jeannerod, M., & Prablanc, C. (1983). The visual control of reaching movements. In J. E. Desmedt (Ed.), *Motor control mechanisms in man* (pp. 13–29). New York: Raven.

Jordan, M. I. (1990). Motor learning and the degrees of freedom problem. In M. Jeannerod (Ed.), *Attention and performance XIII: Motor representation and control* (pp. 796–836). Hillsdale, NJ: Lawrence Erlbaum Associates.

Jordan, M. I., & Rosenbaum, D. A. (1989). Action. In M. I. Posner (Ed.), *Foundations of cognitive science* (pp. 727–768). Cambridge, MA: MIT Press.

Kahneman, D. (1973). *Attention and effort.* Englewood Cliffs, NJ: Prentice-Hall.

Kahneman, D., & Treisman, A. (1984). Changing views of attention and automaticity. In R. Parasuraman & R. Davies (Eds.), *Varieties of attention* (pp. 29–61). New York: Academic Press.

Kalil, R. E., & Freedman, S. J. (1966). Intermanual transfer of compensation for displaced vision. *Perceptual and Motor Skills, 22,* 123–126.

Kausler, D. H. (1974). *Psychology of verbal learning and memory.* New York: Academic press.

Kawato, M., Furukawa, K., & Suzuki, R. (1987). A hierarchical neural-network for control and learning of voluntary movements. *Biological Cybernetics, 57,* 169–185.

Kawato, M., Isobe, M., Maeda, Y., & Suzuki, R. (1988). Coordinates transformation and learning control for visually-guided voluntary movement with iteration: A Newton-like method in a function space. *Biological Cybernetics, 59,* 161–177.

Keele, S. W. (1968). Movement control in skilled motor performance. *Psychological Review, 70,* 387–403.

Keele, S. W. (1981). Behavioral analysis of movement. In V. B. Brooks (Ed.), *Handbook of Physiology, Sec. 1. The nervous system, Vol. 2. Motor control, Pt. 2* (pp. 1391–1414). Baltimore, MD: American Physiological Society.

Keele, S. W. (1986). Motor control. In K. Boff, L. Kaufman, & J. Thomas (Eds.), *Handbook of perception and human performance* (pp. 30.1–30.60). New York: Wiley.

Kelso, J. A. S. (1982). Concepts and issues in human motor behavior: Coming to grips with the jargon. In J. A. S. Kelso (Ed.), *Human motor behavior: An introduction* (pp. 21–58). Hillsdale, NJ: Lawrence Erlbaum Associates.

Kelso, J. A. S., Cook, E., Olson, M. E., & Epstein, W. (1975). Allocation of attention and the locus of adaptation to displaced vision. *Journal of Experimental Psychology, 1,* 237–245.

Kelso, J. A. S., & Kay, B. A. (1987). Information and control: A macroscopic analysis of perception–action coupling. In H. Heuer & A. F. Sanders (Eds.), *Perspectives on perception and action* (pp. 3–32). Hillsdale, NJ: Lawrence Erlbaum Associates.

Kelso, J. A. S., Southard, D. L., & Goodman, D. (1979). On the coordination of two-handed movements. *Journal of Experimental Psychology: Human Perception and Performance, 5,* 229–238.

Kelso, J. A. S., & Wallace, S. A. (1978). Conscious mechanisms in movement. In G. E. Stelmach (Ed.), *Information processing in motor control and learning* (pp. 79–116). New York: Academic Press.

Kennedy, J. M. (1969). Prismatic displacement and the remembered location of targets. *Perception and Psychophysics, 5,* 218–220.

Klein, R. M. (1976). Attention and movement. In G. E. Stelmach (Ed.), *Motor control: Issues and trends* (pp. 143–173). New York: Academic Press.

Koh, K., & Meyer, D. E. (1991). Function learning: Induction of continuous stimulus-response relations. *Journal of Experimental Psychology: Learning, Memory, and Cognition, 17,* 811–836.

Kohler, I. (1964). *Uber Aufbau und Wandlungen der Wahrnehmungswelt* [The formation and transformation of the perceptual world]. (H. Fiss, Trans.). Vienna: Austrian Academy of Science. *Psychological Issues, 3(4),* 1–173. (Original work published 1951)

Kornheiser, A. S. (1976). Adaptation to laterally displaced vision: A review. *Psychological Bulletin, 83,* 783–816.

Kravitz, J. (1972). Conditioned adaptation to prismatic displacement. *Perception and Psychophysics, 11,* 38–42.

Kravitz, J. H., & Wallach, H. (1966). Adaptation to displaced vision contingent upon vibrating stimulation. *Psychonomic Science, 6,* 465–466.

Kupfermann, I. (1981). Localization of higher function. In E. R. Kandel & J. H. Schwartz (Eds.), *Principles of neural science* (pp. 580–592). New York: Elsevier/North-Holland.

Lackner, J. (1973). The role of posture in adaptation to visual rearrangement. *Neuropsychologia, 11,* 33–44.

Larish, J. F., & Flach, J. M. (1990). Source of optical information useful for perception of speed in rectilinear self-motion. *Journal of Experimental Psychology: Human Perception and Performance, 16,* 295–302.

Lashley, K. S. (1930). Basic neural mechanisms in behavior. *Psychological Review, 37,* 1–24.

Lee, D. N. (1980). Visuo-motor coordination in space-time. In G. E. Stelmach & J. Requin (Eds.), *Tutorials in motor behavior* (pp. 281–285). Amsterdam: North-Holland.

Lee, D. N, & Thomson, J. A. (1982). Vision in action: The control of locomotion. In D. J. Ingle, M. A. Goodale, & R. J. W. Mansfield (Eds.), *Analysis of visual behavior* (pp. 411–433). Cambridge, MA: MIT Press.

Lee, T. D., White, M. A., & Carnahan, H. (1990). On the role of knowledge of results in motor learning: Exploring the guidance hypothesis. *Journal of Motor Behavior, 22,* 191–208.

Link, S. W. (1992). *The wave theory of difference and similarity.* Hillsdale, NJ: Lawrence Erlbaum Associates.

Llinás, R., & Pellionisz, A. (1985). Cerebellar function and the adaptive feature of the central nervous system. In A. Berthoz & G. Mevill Jones (Eds.), *Reviews in oculomotor research: Vol. 1. Adaptive mechanisms in gaze control* (pp. 223–231). Amsterdam: Elsevier.

Longuet-Higgins, H. C., & Prazdney, K. (1980). The interpretation of a moving retinal image. *Proceedings of the Royal Society of London B, 208,* 385–397.

Lorenz, K. Z. (1981). *The foundations of ethology.* New York: Springer-Verlag.

MacKay, D. M. (1973). Visual stability and voluntary eye movements. In R. Jung (Ed.), *Handbook of sensory physiology: Central processing of visual information* (Vol. 7, Pt. 3, pp. 307–331). New York: Springer-Verlag.

MacKay, D. M., & Mittelstaedt, M. (1974). Visual stability and motor control (reafference revisited). In W. D. Keidel, W. Handler, & M. Spreng (Eds.), *Kybernetik und Bionik: Cybernetics and Bionics* (pp. 71–79). Munich: Oldenboug.

MacKenzie, C. L., & Marteniuk, R. G. (1985). Motor skill: Feedback, knowledge, and structural issues. *Canadian Journal of Psychology, 39,* 313–337.

Marr, D. (1982). *Vision: A computational investigation into the human representation and processing of visual information.* San Francisco: Freeman.

Marteniuk, R. G. (1992). Issues in goal directed motor learning: Feedforward control, motor equivalence, specificity, and artificial neural networks. In G. E. Stelmach & J. Requin (Eds.), *Tutorials in motor behavior II* (pp. 101–124). Amsterdam: Elsevier Science.

Martin, O., & Prablanc, C. (1992). Online control of hand reaching at undetected target displacements. In G. E. Stelmach & J. Requin (Eds.), *Tutorials in motor behavior II* (pp. 343–355). Amsterdam: Elsevier Science.

Masson, M. E. J. (1991). Cognitive theories of skill acquisition. In R. B. Wilberg (Ed.), *The learning, memory, and perception of perceptual–motor skills* (pp. 15–33). Amsterdam: North- Holland. (Original work published 1990)

Matin, L., Stevens, J. K., & Picoult, E. (1983). Perceptual consequences of experimental extraocular muscle paralysis. In A. Hein & M. Jeannerod (Eds.), *Spatially oriented behavior* (pp. 243–262). New York: Springer-Verlag.

Matthews, P. B. C. (1977). Muscle afferents and kinaesthesia. *British Medical Bulletin, 33,* 137–142.

McCloskey, D. I. (1973). Differences between the sense of movement and position shown by the effects of loading and vibration of muscles in man. *Brain Research, 61,* 119–131.

McCloskey, D. I. (1981). Corollary discharges: Motor commands and perception. In V. B. Brooks (Ed.), *Handbook of physiology: Section 1, The nervous system; Vol. II, Motor control, Part 2* (pp. 1415–1447). Bethesda, MD: American Physiological Society.

McGonigle, B., & Flook, J. (1978). Long-term retention of single and multistate prismatic adaptation by humans. *Nature, 272,* 364–366.

McLaughlin, S. C., & Bower, J. L, (1965). Auditory localization and judgment of straight ahead during adaptation to prism. *Psychonomic Science, 2,* 283–284.

McLaughlin, S. C., & Webster, R. G. (1967). Changes in straight-ahead eye position during adaptation to wedge prisms. *Perception and Psychophysics, 2,* 37–44.

McLeod, P. (1977). A dual task response modality effect: Support for multiprocessor models of attention. *Quarterly Journal of Experimental Psychology, 29,* 651–668.

McLeod, P. (1980). What can RT tell us about the attentional demands of movement? In G. E. Stelmach & J. Requin (Eds.), *Tutorials in motor behavior* (pp. 579–589). Amsterdam: North- Holland.

McMahon, T. A. (1984). *Muscle, reflexes, and locomotion.* Princeton, NJ: Princeton University Press.

Melamed, L. E., Haley, M., & Gildow, J. W. (1973). Effect of external target presence on visual adaptation with active and passive movement. *Journal of Experimental Psychology, 98,* 125–130.

Meyer, D. E., Abrams, R. A., Kornblum, S., Wright, C. E., & Smith, J. E. K. (1988). Optimality in human motor performance: Idea control of rapid aimed movements. *Psychological Review, 95,* 340–370.

Mikaelian, H. H. (1970). Adaptation to rearranged eye–foot coordination. *Perception and Psychophysics, 8,* 222–224.

Mikaelian, H. H. (1972). Lack of bilateral generalization of adaptation to auditory rearrangement. *Perception and Psychophysics, 11,* 222–224.

Mikaelian, H. H. (1974). Adaptation to displaced hearing: A nonproprioceptive change. *Journal of Experimental Psychology, 103,* 326–330.

Mikaelian, H. H. (1990). Adaptation to tilt is not produced by eye-muscle potentiation. *Vision Research, 30,* 779–783.

Mikaelian, H. H., & Held, R. (1964). Two types of adaptation to an optically rotated field. *American Journal of Psychology, 77,* 257–263.

Miller, J., & Festinger, L. (1977). Impact of oculomotor retraining on the visual perception of curvature. *Journal of Experimental Psychology: Human Perception and Performance, 3,* 187–200.

Milner, A. D., & Goodale, M. A. (1993). Visual pathways to perception and action. In T. P. Hicks, S. Molotchnikoff, & T. Ono (Eds.), *The visually responsive neuron: From basic neurophysiology to behavior* (pp. 317–337). Amsterdam: Elsevier.

Mishkin, M. (1993). Cerebral memory circuits. In T. A. Poggio & D. A. Glaser (Eds.), *Exploring brain functions: Models in Neuroscience* (pp. 113–125). New York: Wiley.

Morasso, P. (1981). Spatial control of arm movements. *Experimental Brain Research, 42,* 223–227.

Newell, K. M. (1976). Knowledge of results and motor learning. In J. Keogh & R. S. Hutton (Eds.), *Exercise and sport science reviews* (pp. 195–228). Santa Barbara, CA: Journal Publishing Affiliates.

Paap, K. R., & Ebenholtz, S. M. (1976). Perceptual consequences of potentiation in extraocular muscles: An alternative explanation for adaptation to wedge prisms. *Journal of Experimental Psychology: Human Perception and Performance, 2,* 457–468.

Paap, K. R., & Ebenholtz, S. M. (1977). Concomitant direction and distance aftereffects of sustained convergence: A muscle potentiation explanation for eye-specific adaptation. *Perception and Psychophysics, 21,* 307–314.

Paillard, J. (1980). The multichanneling of visual cues and the organization of visually guided response. In G. E. Stelmach & J. Requin (Eds.), *Tutorials in motor behavior* (pp. 259–279). New York: North-Holland.

Paillard, J. (1982). The contribution of peripheral and central vision to visually guided reaching. In D. J. Ingle, M. A. Goodale, & R. J. W. Mansfield (Eds.), *Analysis of visual behavior* (pp. 367–385). Cambridge, MA: MIT Press.

Paillard, J. (1991a). Knowing where and knowing how to get there. In J. Paillard (Ed.), *Brain and space* (pp. 461–482). New York: Oxford University Press.

Paillard, J. (1991b). Motor and representational framing of space. In J. Paillard (Ed.), *Brain and space* (pp. 163–184). New York: Oxford University Press.

Paillard, J., Jordon, P., & Brouchon, M. (1981). Visual motion cues to prismatic adaptation: Evidence of two separate and additive processes. *Acta Psychologica, 48,* 253–270.

Pellionisz, A. (1984). Coordination: A vector-matrix description of overcomplete CNS coordinates and a tensorial solution using the Moore-Penrose generalized inverse. *Journal of Theoretical Biology, 110,* 353–376.

Pellionisz, A. (1985). Tensorial aspects of the multidimensional approach to the vestibulo-oculomotor reflex and gaze. In A. Berthoz, & G. Mevill Jones (Eds.), *Reviews in oculomotor research: Vol. 1. Adaptive mechanisms in gaze control* (pp. 281–296). Amsterdam: Elsevier.

Pellionisz, A., & Llinás, R. (1985). Tensor network theory of the metaorganization of functional geometries in the central nervous system. *Neuroscience, 16,* 245–273.

Pew, R. W. (1966). Acquisition of hierarchical control over the temporal organization of a skill. *Journal of Experimental Psychology, 71,* 764–761.

Pick, H. L., Jr., & Hay, J. C. (1965). A passive test of the Held reafference hypothesis. *Perceptual and Motor Skills, 20,* 1070–1072.

Polit, A., & Bizzi, E. (1978). Processes controlling arm movements in monkeys. *Science, 201,* 1235–1237.

Posner, M. I., & Keele, S. W. (1969). Attention demands of movement. *Proceedings of the 16th International Conference of Applied Psychology* (pp. 412–422). Amsterdam: Swets & Zeitlinger.

Posner, M. I., & Snyder, C. R. R. (1975). Attention and cognitive control. In R. L. Solso (Ed.), *Information processing and cognition* (pp. 55–86). Hillsdale, NJ: Lawrence Erlbaum Associates.

Poulton, E. C. (1957). On prediction in skilled movements. *Psychological Bulletin, 54,* 467–478.

Prablanc, C., Echallier, J. F., Jeannerod, M., & Komilis, E. (1979). Optimal response of eye and hand motor systems in pointing at a visual target. II. Static and dynamic visual cues in the control of hand movement. *Biological Cybernetics, 35,* 183–187.

Prablanc, C., Echallier, J. F., Komilis, E., & Jeannerod, M. (1979). Optimal response of eye and hand motor systems in pointing at a visual target: I. Spatiotemporal characteristics of eye and hand movements and their relationships with varying the among of visual information. *Biological Cybernetics, 35,* 113–124.

Proteau, L. (1992). On the specificity of learning and the role of visual information for movement control. In L. Proteau & D. Elliott (Eds.), *Vision and motor control* (pp. 67–103). Amsterdam: Elsevier Science Publishers.

Radeau, M. (1994). Auditory–visual spatial interaction and modularity. *Cahiers de Psychologie/Current Psychology of Cognition, 13,* 3–51.

Radeau, M., & Bertelson, P. (1977). Adaptation to auditory-visual discordance and ventriloquism in semirealistic situations. *Perception and Psychophysics, 22,* 137–146.

Radeau, M., & Bertelson, P. (1978). Cognitive factors and adaptation to auditory–visual discordance. *Perception and Psychophysics, 23,* 341–343.

Rader, S. D. (1989). *The effects of target availability and cognitive load on prism adaptation during eye–hand coordination.* Unpublished master's thesis, Illinois State University, Normal.

Redding, G. M. (1973a). Simultaneous visual adaptation to tilt and displacement: A test of independent processes. *Bulletin of the Psychonomic Society, 2,* 41–42.

Redding, G. M. (1973b). Visual adaptation to tilt and displacement: Same or different processes? *Perception and Psychophysics, 14,* 193–200.

Redding, G. M. (1975a). Decay of visual adaptation to tilt and displacement. *Perception and Psychophysics, 17,* 203–208.

Redding, G. M. (1975b). Simultaneous visuo-motor adaptation to optical tilt and displacement. *Perception and Psychophysics, 17,* 97–100.

Redding, G. M. (1978). Additivity in adaptation to optical tilt. *Journal of Experimental Psychology: Human Perception and Performance, 4,* 178–190.

Redding, G. M. (1979). Attention as an explanatory concept in perceptual adaptation. *Behavioral and Brain Sciences* (commentary), *2,* 77–78.

Redding, G. M. (1981). Effects of homogeneous and variable exposure on adaptation to optical tilt. *Journal of Experimental Psychology: Human Perception and Performance, 7,* 130–140.

Redding, G. M., Clark, S. E., & Wallace, B. (1985). Attention and prism adaptation. *Cognitive Psychology, 17,* 1–25.

Redding, G. M., Rader, S. D., & Lucas, D. R. (1992). Cognitive load and prism adaptation. *Journal of Motor Behavior, 24,* 238–246.

Redding, G. M., & Wallace, B. (1976). Components of displacement adaptation in acquisition and decay as a function of hand and hall exposure. *Perception and Psychophysics, 20,* 453–459.

Redding, G. M., & Wallace, B. (1978). Sources of "overadditivity" in prism adaptation. *Perception and Psychophysics, 24,* 58–62.

Redding, G. M., & Wallace, B. (1985a). Cognitive interference in prism adaptation. *Perception and Psychophysics, 37,* 225–230.

Redding, G. M., & Wallace, B. (1985b). Perceptual–motor coordination and adaptation during locomotion: Determinants of prism adaptation in hall exposure. *Perception and Psychophysics, 38,* 320–330.

Redding, G. M., & Wallace, B. (1987). Perceptual–motor coordination and prism adaptation during locomotion: A control for head posture contributions. *Perception and Psychophysics, 42,* 269–274.

Redding, G. M., & Wallace, B. (1988a). Adaptive mechanisms in perceptual–motor coordination: Components of prism adaptation. *Journal of Motor Behavior, 20,* 242–254.

Redding, G. M., & Wallace, B. (1988b). Components of prism adaptation in terminal and concurrent exposure: Organization of the eye–hand coordination loop. *Perception and Psychophysics, 44,* 59–68.

Redding, G. M., & Wallace, B. (1988c). Head posture effects in prism adaptation during hallway exposure. *Perception and Psychophysics, 44,* 69–75.

Redding, G. M., & Wallace, B. (1990). Effects on prism adaptation of duration and timing of visual feedback during pointing. *Journal of Motor Behavior, 22,* 209–224.

Redding, G. M., & Wallace, B. (1992a). Adaptive eye–hand coordination: Implications of prism adaptation for perceptual–motor organization. In L. Proteau & D. Elliott (Eds.), *Vision and motor control* (pp. 105–127). Amsterdam: Elsevier.

Redding, G. M., & Wallace, B. (1992b). Effects of pointing rate and availability of visual feedback on visual and proprioceptive components of prism adaptation. *Journal of Motor Behavior, 24,* 226–237.

Redding, G. M., & Wallace, B. (1993). Adaptive coordination and alignment of eye and hand. *Journal of Motor Behavior, 25,* 75–88.

Redding, G. M., & Wallace, B. (1994). Effects of movement duration and visual feedback on visual and proprioceptive components of prism adaptation. *Journal of Motor Behavior, 26,* 257–266.

Redding, G. M., & Wallace, B. (1995a). Contributions of motor control and spatial alignment to prism adaptation. In B. G. Bardy, R. J. Bootsma, & Y. Guiard (Eds.), *Studies in perception and action III* (pp. 277–280). Hillsdale, NJ: Lawrence Erlbaum Associates.

Redding, G. M., & Wallace, B. (1995b, November). *Prism adaptation during ball throwing.* Paper presented at the 36th annual meeting of the Psychonomic Society, Los Angeles, CA.

Redding, G. M., & Wallace, B. (1996a). Adaptive spatial alignment and strategic perceptual–motor control. *Journal of Experimental Psychology: Human Perception and Performance, 22,* 379–394.

Redding G. M., & Wallace, B. (1996b, in press). Prism adaptation during target pointing from visible and nonvisible starting locations. *Journal of Motor Behavior.*

Rieser, J. J., Pick, H. L., Jr., Ashmead, D. H., & Garing, A. E. (1995). Calibration of human locomotion and models of perceptual–motor organization. *Journal of Experimental Psychology: Human Perception and Performance, 21,* 480–497.

Robinson, D. A. (1975). A quantitative analysis of extraocular muscle cooperation and squint. *Investigations in Opthalmology, 14,* 801–825.

Robinson, D. A. (1976). Adaptive gain control of vestibulo-ocular reflex by the cerebellum. *Journal of Neurophysiology, 39,* 954–969.

Robinson, D. A. (1982). The use of matrices in analyzing the three-dimensional behavior of the vestibulo-ocular reflex. *Biological Cybernetics, 46,* 53–66.

Robinson, D. A. (1985). The coordinates of neurons in the vestibulo-ocular reflex. In A. Berthoz & G. Mevill Jones (Eds.), *Reviews in oculomotor research: Vol. 1. Adaptive mechanisms in gaze control* (pp. 297–311). Amsterdam: Elsevier.

Rock, I. (1966). *The nature of perceptual adaptation.* New York: Basic Books.

Rock, I., & Harris, C. S. (1967). Vision and touch. *Scientific American, 216,* 96–104.

Romack, J. L., Buss, R. A., & Bingham, G. P. (1992). "Adaptation" to displacement prisms is sensorimotor learning. In J. K. Kruschke (Ed.), *Proceedings of the 14th Annual*

Conference of the Cognitive Science Society (pp. 1080–1085). Hillsdale, NJ: Lawrence Erlbaum Associates.

Rosenbaum, D. A. (1980). Human movement initiation: Specification of arm, direction, and extent. *Journal of Experimental Psychology: Human Perception and Performance, 109,* 4, 444–474.

Rossetti, Y., & Koga, K. (1994). *Visual–proprioceptive discrepancy and motor control: Modification of fast-pointing trajectories during prismatic displacement of vision.* Unpublished manuscript.

Rossetti, Y., Desmurget, M., & Prablanc, C. (1995). Vectorial coding of movement: Vision, proprioception, or both? *Journal of Neurophysiology, 74*(1), 457–463.

Rossetti, Y., Koga, S., & Mano, T. (1993). Prismatic displacement of vision induces transient changes in the timing of eye–hand coordination. *Perception and Psychophysics, 54,* 355–364.

Rossetti, Y., Stelmach, G., Desmurget, M., Prablanc, C., & Jeannerod, M. (1994). The effect of viewing the static hand prior to movement onset on pointing kinematics and variability. *Experimental Brain Research, 101,* 323–330.

Rozin, P. (1976). The evaluation of intelligence and access to the cognitive unconscious. In J. A. Sprague & A. N. Epstein (Eds.), *Progress in Psychobiology and Physiological Psychology* (Vol. 6, pp. 245–280). New York: Academic Press.

Rozin, P., & Schull, J. (1988). The adaptive-evolutionary point of view in experimental psychology. In R. C. Atkinson, R. J. Herrnstein, G. Lindzey, & R. D. Luce (Eds.), *Handbook of experimental psychology: Vol. 1. Perception and motivation* (pp. 503–546). New York: Wiley.

Salmoni, A. W., Schmidt, R. A., & Walter, C. B. (1984). Knowledge of results and motor learning: A review and critical reappraisal. *Psychological Bulletin, 95,* 355–386.

Salomi, A. W., Sullivan, S. J., & Starkes, J. L. (1976). The attention demands of movement: A critique of the probe technique. *Journal of Motor Behavior, 8,* 161–169.

Saltzman, E. L. (1979). Levels of sensorimotor representation. *Journal of Mathematical Psychology, 20,* 91–163.

Schmidt, R. A. (1975). A schema theory of discrete motor skill learning. *Psychological Review, 82,* 225–260.

Schmidt, R. A. (1976). Control processes in motor skills. *Exercise and Sport Sciences Review, 4,* 229–261.

Schmidt, R. A. (1987). The acquisition of skill: Some modifications to the perception–action relationship through practice. In H. Heuer & A. F. Sanders (Eds.), *Perspectives on perception and action* (pp. 77–103). Hillsdale, NJ: Lawrence Erlbaum Associates.

Schmidt, R. A. (1988). *Motor control and learning* (2nd ed.). Champaign, IL: Human Kinetics.

Schmidt, R. A., & McGown, C. (1980). Terminal accuracy of unexpectedly loaded rapid movements: Evidence for a mass-spring mechanism in programming. *Journal of Motor Behavior, 12,* 149–161.

Schmidt, R. A., Zelaznik, H. N., Hawkins, B., Frank, J. S., & Quinn, J. T., Jr. (1979). Motor output variability: A theory for the accuracy of rapid motor acts. *Psychological Review, 86,* 415–451.

Schneider, W., Dumais, S. T., & Shiffrin, R. M. (1984). Automatic and control processing and attention. In R. Parasuraman and R. Davies (Eds.), *Varieties of attention* (pp. 1–27). New York: Academic Press.

Schneider, W., & Fisk, A. D. (1983). Attention theory and mechanisms for skilled perform-ance. In R. Magill (Ed.), *Memory and control of action* (pp 119–143). New York: North-Holland.

Schneider, W., & Shiffrin, R. M. (1977a). Automatic and controlled information processing in vision. In D. LaBerge & S. J. Samuels (Eds.), *Basic processes in reading* (pp. 127–154). Hillsdale, NJ: Lawrence Erlbaum Associates.

Schneider, W., & Shiffrin, R. (1977b). Controlled and automatic human information proc-essing: I. Detection, search, and attention. *Psychological Review, 84,* 1–66.

Schwartz, A. B., Kettner, R. E., & Georgopoulos, A. P. (1988). Primate motor cortex and free arm movements to visual targets in three-dimensional space: I. Relations between single cell discharge and direction of movement. *Journal of Neuroscience, 8,* 2913–2927.

Segal, S. J., & Fusella, V. (1970). Influence of imagining pictures and sounds on detection of visual and auditory signals. *Journal of Experimental Psychology, 83,* 458–464.

Shepard, R. N. (1981). Psychophysical complementarity. In M. Kobovy & J. R. Pomerantz (Eds.), *Perceptual organization* (pp. 279–341). Hillsdale, NJ: Lawrence Erlbaum Asso-ciates.

Shepard, R. N. (1984). Ecological constraints on internal representation: Resonant kinemat-ics of perceiving, imagining, thinking, and dreaming. *Psychological Review, 91,* 417–447.

Shepard, R. N. (1989). Internal representation of universal regularities: A challenge for connectionism. In L. Nadel, L. A. Cooper, P. Culicover, & R. M. Harish (Eds.), *Neural connections, mental computation* (pp. 104–134). Cambridge, MA: MIT Press.

Shepard, R. N. (1990). *Mind sights.* New York: Freeman.

Sherrington, C. S. (1918). Observations on the sensual role of the proprioceptive nerve supply of the extrinsic ocular muscles. *Brain, 41,* 332–343.

Shiffrin, R., & Schneider, W. (1977). Controlled and automatic human information process-ing: II. Perceptual learning, automatic attending, and a general theory. *Psychological Review, 84,* 128–190.

Shiffrin, R. M., & Dumais, S. T. (1981). The development of automatism. In J. R. Anderson (Ed.), *Cognitive skills and their acquisition* (pp. 111–140). Hillsdale, NJ: Lawrence Erlbaum Associates.

Simpson, J. I., & Graf, W. (1985). The selection of reference frames by nature and its investigation. In A. Berthoz & G. Mevill Jones (Eds.), *Reviews in oculomotor research: Vol. 1. Adaptive mechanisms in gaze control* (pp. 3–16). Amsterdam: Elsevier.

Singer, G., & Day, R. H. (1966). Spatial adaptation and aftereffect with optically transformed vision: Effects of active and passive responding and the relationship between test and exposure responses. *Journal of Experimental Psychology, 71,* 725–731.

Skavenski, A. A. (1972). Inflow as a source of extraretinal eye position information. *Vision Research, 12,* 221–229.

Skavenski, A. A., Haddad, G., & Steinman, R. M. (1972). The extraretinal signal for the visual perception of direction. *Perception and Psychophysics, 11,* 287–290.

Slotnick, R. A. (1969). Adaptation to curvature distortion. *Journal of Experimental Psychol-ogy, 81,* 441–448.

Smith, W. M., & Bowen, K. F. (1980). The effects of delayed and displaced visual feedback on motor control. *Journal of Motor Behavior, 12,* 91–101.

Soechting, J. F. (1989). Elements of coordinated arm movements in three-dimensional space. In S. A. Wallace (Ed.), *Perspectives on the coordination of movement* (pp. 47–83). Amsterdam: North Holland.

Soechting, J. F., & Flanders, M. (1989). Errors in pointing are due to approximations in sensorimotor transformations. *Journal of Neurophysiology, 62,* 595–608.

Soechting, J. F., & Lacquaniti, F. (1981). Invariant characteristics of a pointing movement in man. *Journal of Neuroscience, 1,* 710–720.

Soechting, J. F., & Terzuolo, C. A. (1990). Sensorimotor transformations and the kinematics of arm movements in three-dimensional space. In M. Jeannerod (Ed.), *Attention and performance XII: Motor representation and control* (pp. 479–494). Hillsdale, NJ: Lawrence Erlbaum Associates.

Sparks, D. L. (1988). Neural cartography: Sensory and motor maps in the superior colliculus. *Brain, Behavior, and Evolution, 31,* 49–56.

Spelke, E. S. (1990). Principles of object perception. *Cognitive Science, 14,* 29–56.

Spelke, E. S., Breinlinger, K., Macomber, J., & Jacobson, K. (1992). Origins of knowledge. *Psychological Review, 99,* 605–632.

Stelmach, G. E. (1982). Information-processing framework for understanding human motor behavior. In J. A. S. Kelso (Ed.), *Human motor behavior: An introduction,* (pp. 93–115). Hillsdale, NJ: Lawrence Erlbaum Associates.

Stillings, N. A., Feinstein, M. H., Garfield, J. L., Rissland, E. L., Rosenbaum, D. A., Weisler, S. E., & Baker-Ward, L. (1987). *Cognitive science: An introduction.* Cambridge, MA: MIT Press.

Stratton, G. M. (1896). Some preliminary experiments on vision without inversion of the retinal image. *Psychological Review, 3,* 611–617.

Stratton, G. M. (1897a). Upright vision and the retinal image. *Psychological Review, 4,* 182–187.

Stratton, G. M. (1897b). Vision without inversion of the retinal image. *Psychological Review, 4,* 341–360, 463–481.

Szentágothai, J, & Arbib, M. A. (1975). *Conceptual models of neural organization.* Cambridge, MA: MIT Press.

Taylor, J. G. (1962). *The behavioral basis of perception.* New Haven, CT: Yale University Press.

Templeton, W. B., Howard, I. P., & Lowman, A. E. (1966). Passively generated adaptation to prismatic distortion. *Perceptual and Motor Skills, 22,* 140–142.

Templeton, W. B., Howard, I. P., & Wilkinson, D. A. (1974). Additivity of components of prismatic adaptation. *Perception and Psychophysics, 15,* 249–257.

Thomson, J. A. (1983). Is continuous visual monitoring necessary in visually guided locomotion? *Journal of Experimental Psychology: Human Perception and Performance, 9,* 427–443.

Treisman, A. (1985). Preattentive processing in vision. *Computer Vision, Graphics, and Image Processing, 31,* 156–177.

Treisman, A. (1992). Perceiving and re-perceiving objects. *American Psychologist, 47,* 862–875.

Tuller, B., Turvey, M. T., & Fitch, H. L. (1982). The Bernstein perspective: II. The concept of muscle linkage or coordinative structure. In J. A. S. Kelso (Ed.), *Human motor behavior: An introduction* (pp. 253–270). Hillsdale, NJ: Lawrence Erlbaum Associates.

Turvey, M. T. (1990). Coordination. *American Psychologist, 45,* 938–953.

Uhlarik, J. J. (1973). Role of cognitive factors on adaptation to prismatic displacement. *Journal of Experimental Psychology, 98,* 223–232.

Uhlarik, J. J., & Canon, L. K. (1971). Influence of concurrent and terminal exposure conditions on the nature of perceptual adaptation. *Journal of Experimental Psychology, 9,* 233–239.

Ungerleider, L. G., & Mishkin, M. (1982). Two cortical systems. In D. J. Ingle, M. A. Goodale, & R. J. W. Mansfield (Eds.), *Analysis of visual behavior* (pp. 549–586). Cambridge, MA: MIT Press.

Uno, Y., Kawato, M., & Suzuki, R. (1989). Formation and control of optimal trajectory in human multijoint arm movements. *Biological Cybernetics, 61,* 89–101.

Wallace, B. (1977). Stability of Wilkinson's model of prism adaptation over time for various targets. *Perception, 6,* 145–151.

Wallace, B., & Garrett, J. B. (1973). Reduced felt arm sensation effects on visual adaptation. *Perception and Psychophysics, 14,* 175–177.

Wallace, B., & Garrett, J. B. (1975). Perceptual adaptation with selective reductions of felt sensation. *Perception, 4,* 437–445.

Wallace, B., & Redding, G. M. (1979). Additivity in prism adaptation as manifested in intermanual and interocular transfer. *Perception and Psychophysics, 25,* 133–136.

Wallach, H. (1968). Informational discrepancy as a basis of perceptual adaptation. In S. J. Freedman (Ed.), *The neuropsychology of spatially oriented behavior* (pp. 209–229). Homewood, IL: Dorsey.

Wallach, H., Moore, M. E., & Davidson, L. (1963). Modification of stereoscopic depth-perception. *American Journal of Psychology, 76,* 191–204.

Webster, R. G. (1969). The relationship between cognitive, motor-kinesthetic, and oculo-motor adaptation. *Perception and Psychophysics, 6,* 33–38.

Weinstein, S., Sersen, E. A., & Weinstein, D. S. (1964). An attempt to replicate a study of disarranged eye–hand coordination. *Perceptual and Motor Skills, 18,* 629–632.

Welch, R. B. (1969). Adaptation to prism-displaced vision: The importance of target pointing. *Perception and Psychophysics, 5,* 305–309.

Welch, R. B. (1971a). Discriminative conditioning of prism adaptation. *Perception and Psychophysics, 10,* 90–92.

Welch, R. B. (1971b). Prism adaptation: The "target-pointing effect" as a function of exposure trials. *Perception and Psychophysics, 9,* 102–104.

Welch, R. B. (1974). Speculations on a model of prism adaptation. *Perception, 3,* 451–460.

Welch, R. B. (1978). *Perceptual modification: Adapting to altered sensory environments.* New York: Academic Press.

Welch, R. B. (1986). Adaptation of space perception. In K. R. Boff, L. Kaufman, & J. R. Thomas (Eds.), *Handbook of perception and human performance, Vol. 1: Sensory processes and perception* (pp. 24.1–24.45). New York: Wiley.

Welch, R. B. (1994). The dissection of intersensory bias: Weighting for Radeau. *Cahiers de Psychologie/Current Psychology of Cognition, 13,* 117–123.

Welch, R. B., & Abel, M. R. (1970). The generality of the "target-pointing effect" in prism adaptation. *Psychonomic Science, 20,* 226–227.

Welch, R. B., Bridgeman, B., Anand, S., & Browman, K. (1991, November). *The acquisition of "dual adaptations" and "adaptation sets."* Paper presented at the 32nd Annual Meeting of the Psychonomic Society, San Franciso, CA.

Welch, R. B., Bridgeman, B., Anand, S., & Browman, K. (1993). Alternating prism exposure causes dual adaptation and generalization to a novel displacement. *Perception and Psychophysics, 54,* 195–204.

Welch, R. B., Choe, C. S., & Heinrich, D. R. (1974). Evidence for a three-component model of prism adaptation. *Journal of Experimental Psychology, 103,* 700–705.

Welch, R. B., & Rhoades, R. W. (1969). The manipulation of informational feedback and its effects upon prism adaptation. *Canadian Journal of Psychology, 23,* 415–428.

Welch, R. B., & Warren, D. H. (1980). Immediate perceptual response to intersensory discrepancy. *Psychological Bulletin, 88,* 638–667.

Welch, R. B., & Warren, D. H. (1986). Intersensory interactions. In K. R. Boff, L. Kaufman, & J. R. Thomas (Eds.), *Handbook of perception and human performance, Vol. 1: Sensory processes and perception* (pp. 25.1–25.36). New York: Wiley.

Welch, R. B., Widawski, M. H., Harrington, J., & Warren, D. H. (1979). An examination of the relationship between visual capture and prism adaptation. *Perception and Psychophysics, 25,* 126–132.

Wilkinson, D. A. (1971). Visual–motor control loop: A linear system? *Journal of Experimental Psychology, 89,* 250–257.

Woodworth, R. S. (1899). The accuracy of voluntary movements. *Psychological Review, Monograph Supplement 3,* Whole No. 114.

Young, D. E., & Schmidt, R. A. (1990). Units of motor behavior: Modifications with practice and feedback. In M. Jeannerod (Ed.), *Attention and performance XIII: Motor representation and control* (pp. 763–795). Hillsdale, NJ: Lawrence Erlbaum Associates.

AUTHOR INDEX

A

Abbs, J. H., 6, 10, 12, 15, 41, 91
Abel, M. R., 57, 112
Abend, W. M., 22
Abrams, R. A., 13, 14, 73, 158
Adams, J. A., 40, 42
Almdale, D. P. J., 6
Anand, S., 83, 166
Anderson, J. R., 39
Annett, J., 143
Anstis, T., 57, 101
Arbib, M. A., 75, 76, 91
Ashmead, D. H., 129
Auerbach, C., 87

B

Bahrick, H. P., 40
Baily, J. S., 57, 111, 112, 118, 149, 152
Baker-Ward, L., 36
Bamber, D., 94, 95, 116
Bardy, B. G., 157
Barr, C. C., 63
Basmajian, J. V., 10
Bauer, J., 105
Beaubaton, D., 11
Beckett, P. A., 112
Bedford, F., 30, 32, 33, 34, 35, 36, 38, 45, 46, 47, 48, 53, 54, 84, 111, 118, 165, 166
Beggs, W. D. A., 143
Berkenblit, M. B., 5, 12, 13
Bernard, E. E., 109
Bernstein, N., 5, 76
Bertelson, P., 53, 136
Biederman, I., 34, 47, 87
Biguer, B., 5, 21, 24, 76
Bingham, G. P., 83, 166

C

Bizzi, E., 5, 13, 14, 22
Bonnet, M., 73
Bootsma, R. J., 157
Bossom, J., 54, 57, 111, 118
Bowen, K. F., 149
Bower, J. L., 53
Breinlinger, K., 34
Bridgeman, B., 83, 166
Briggs, G. E., 40
Brouchon, M., 60, 76
Browman, K. E., 83, 166
Buchanan, T. S., 6
Bullock, D., 5, 6, 13, 14, 15, 45, 49, 54, 72, 73, 74, 91
Burnham, C. A., 94, 95, 116
Buss, R. A., 83

Callan, J. W., 118, 119
Caminiti, R., 73
Canon, L. K., 9, 62, 63, 96, 115, 141, 146, 147
Carey, D. P., 54
Carlton, L. G., 10, 15
Carnahan, H., 83
Carson, R. G., 90
Casey, A., 37
Cattell, J. M., 13
Choe, C. S., 61, 106, 112, 163
Chua, R., 90
Churchland, P. S., 28, 67, 87
Clark, S. E., 63, 116, 129, 135, 150
Cohen, H. B., 141
Cohen, M. M., 141
Cole, K. J., 6, 10, 15, 41, 91
Cook, E., 9, 62, 115, 116
Coren, S., 57, 112
Craske, B., 28, 48, 63, 65, 88, 101, 103, 104, 105, 111, 112

SUBJECT INDEX